Journal of The American Academy of Psychotherapists

VOICES

THE ART AND SCIENCE OF PSYCHOTHERAPY

In treasured memory of Tom Burns (1951-2024)

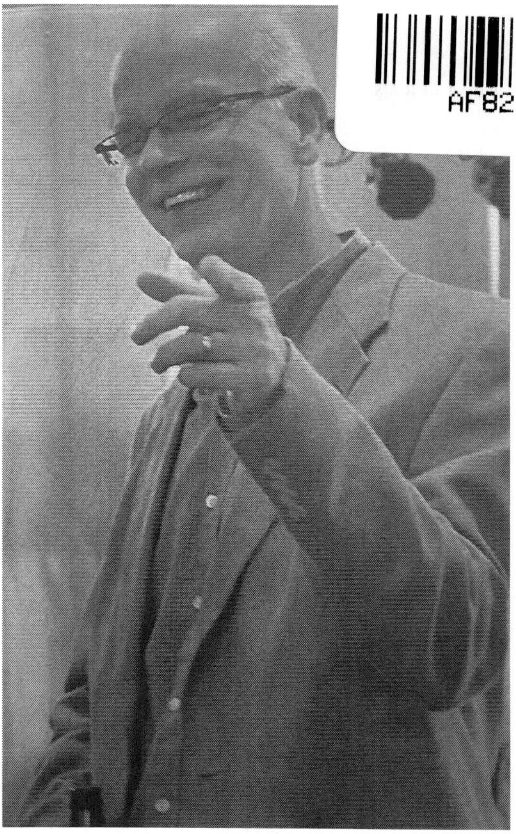

One cannot individuate without being with other human beings. One cannot individuate on top of Mt. Everest or in a cave somewhere where one doesn't see people for seventy years: one can only individuate with or against something or somebody. Being an individual is always a link in the chain.

—*Carl Jung*

Founded in 1964 by John Warkentin, PhD, MD and Thomas Leland, MD

Voices: *Journal of the American Academy of Psychotherapists*

Special thanks:
Jennifer Baumann for permission to use photographs titled "State Theatre" and "Empty Train"
Piero Bonamico for producing the audio file that accompanies *"Small Things Like These."*

Cover:

Jonathan Borofsky, Digital Man, 2016, 24' tall, painted steel.
Courtesy of the Center for Maine Contemporary Art, photo by Dave Clough

Published one time per year.
Design and Production by Kim Leaird

AAP Web Site: www.aapweb.com

VOICES: THE ART AND SCIENCE OF PSYCHOTHERAPY (ISSN 0042-8272) is published by the American Academy of Psychotherapists.

The Executive Director of AAP is LeAnna Hamer and her email address for all business inquiries (subscriptions, change of address, etc.) is: aapexecdirector@gmail.com, or check the Voices menu at AAPweb.com. The postal address for AAP is: P.O. Box 3220, Kingsport, TN 37664.

Journal of the American Academy of Psychotherapists

VOICES

THE ART AND SCIENCE OF PSYCHOTHERAPY

Links in the Chain: Tradition and Change in Psychotherapy 2025: Volume 61

Voices: Journal of the American Academy of Psychotherapists		i
Table of Contents		v
Editorial		
Links in the Chain	Editorial Team	1
Articles		
Way Up in the Parent-Filled Bleachers	Tom Burns	3
Out of Bounds	Lisa Zimmerman	5
Commentary	Stephanie Spalding	10
The Therapy of Allowance, or Master's Degree in Anything	Svetlana Kreimer	11
Commentary	Molly Donovan	17
What Do Young Therapists Want?	Doris Jackson	19
	Camilla Dorment	20
	Marvice Marcus	21
	Aaron Severn	22
	Hilary Hla	23
	Alec Addleton	24
Becoming a Play Therapist	Penelope Norton	25
Necessity is the Mother of Invention	Kim Rust	32
Commentary	Z Rosenzweig	36
Commentary	Matthew Leary	37
Dr. Elvin Semrad: A Memorable Teacher	Jerry Gans	43
Commentary	Jonathan Farber	48
A Song of Appreciation	Barry Wepman	49
Commentary	Abby MacDonald	52
Commentary	Peggy Brooks	53
Questions and Contradictions: Mentoring and the Psychotherapy Relationship	Jonathan Farber	55
The Art of Psychotherapy and the Psychotherapy of Art	Avrum G. Weiss	63
Of Pens and Swords	Sylvia Flescher	71
Selling Bliss	Matthew Varley	73
Commentary	Rona Engels	77
Commentary	Stephanie Spalding	77

Developing the Person of the Therapist—A Tradition Taught Through the Stories We Tell	Marilyn Schwartz	80
A Psychologist Looks Back	Edward H. Jacobs	85
Healing Through Poetry	David S. Ribner	91
Treating a Dying Patient– Flying the Plane and "The New Horizon"	Judith Logue	103
Mentoring Moments		
Turtles	Campbell States	111
By the Way	Penelope Norton	112
For Good	Ann Reifman	113
Looking Back	Hallie Lovett	115
A Therapist Learns to Keep His Mouth Shut	Murray Scher	116
Finding AAP	John Rhead	117
Poetry		
This, Last Swallow, Sorrows	Katherine Williams	39
Morning Paper (November 6, 2024), Speechless	Tom Large	78
Reviews		
Movie: Thunderbolts	Ezra Farber	119
Movie: Emilia Pérez	Bob Schulte	121
Book and Movie: Small Things Like These	Erin McCarthy	124
Images		
Train	Jennifer Baumann	2
Doors	Molly Donovan	18
Passing Through	Molly Donovan	42
African Antelopes	Fern Bleu	66
Winter on the Farm	David Pellegrini	68
Pathway	Molly Donovan	86
Sitting on a Bench	Iftikhar Alam	102
Links in the Chain	Molly Donovan	110
State Theatre	Jennifer Baumann	118
Voices		
Subscribe to Voices		128
Guidelines for Contributors		125
The American Academy of Psychotherapists		126

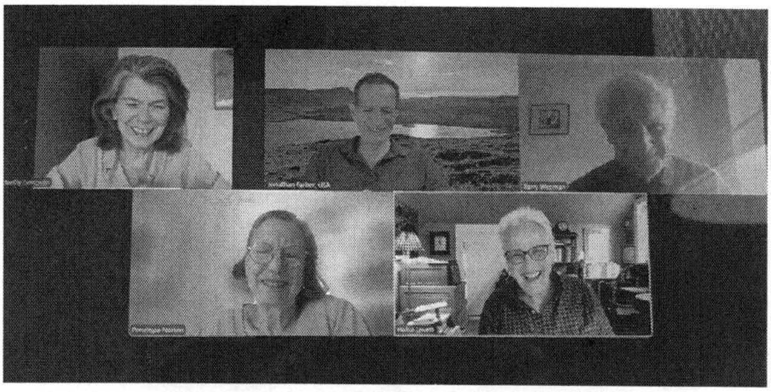

Editorial

Links in the Chain

WE WERE A GROUP OF SIX WHEN WE WERE SUMMONED DOWN FROM OUR COMFORTABLE PERCH ON THE *VOICES* MASTHEAD, AND FOUND OURSELVES AGREEING TO TAKE ON THE MISSION OF PRODUCING THIS SINGLE ISSUE OF *VOICES 2025.* We have each been grateful for the ways in which *Voices* has touched our lives over the years—whether because it brought us to the Academy, provided us with printed mentoring and inspiration, or because it mirrored our struggles as therapists—and we each felt the need to support the journal .

To our deep sorrow, one of the first challenges we had to face was the loss of one of us, Tom Burns, who conceived this project. Tom's passion for *Voices,* his gifts as a writer and editor, along with his humor—creative, playful, and sometimes dry but always warm and sensitive—pulled us into what we knew would be a lot of work. What got the remaining five of us through was working with each of the others: Hallie, Pennie, Jon, Molly and Barry. United in our wish for *Voices* to continue, this collaboration deepened our connections to each other, and our appreciation for each other's singular talents and life energies. As a group of senior therapists, we feel the importance in investing in future generations of therapists, as a means to a sense of purpose for ourselves, or, as a means of returning or "giving back," the richness we received from our own mentors and elders in the profession. This *Voices* issue is another link in a chain of issues that began before some of our members' parents were born, and it is fitting that we dedicate this one to the memory of Tom Burns, since his spirit has been with us throughout our work together, and since the theme of this issue looks back to our collective professional history, and forward to our future.

As a team, we share a celebration of the written word as well as the mission of *Voices* to present the the work of psychotherapy in its fullness: the transactions with the patients, and the inner experience of the therapist. With the many changes in the world and technology, the human to human relationship remains the bedrock of the work where people come to know themselves more fully, and the astonishing power of depth psychotherapy is needed more than ever to remind us humans who we are and of the potentials we have.

In presenting this particular issue to you, we hope we have carried on the tradition of psychotherapists mentoring one another, and we hope we have done so in a creative spirit that honors Tom's memory. We imagine that if he observed some of our "mentoring moments" along the way—some of our heated debates, or clumsy miscommunications—he would have more than a few laughs, and we imagine he would read this issue with approval. We hope you find it worth your time and attention.

—Editors: Molly Donovan, PhD; Jonathan Farber, PhD; Hallie Lovett, PhD; Penelope Norton, PhD; and Barry Wepman, PhD

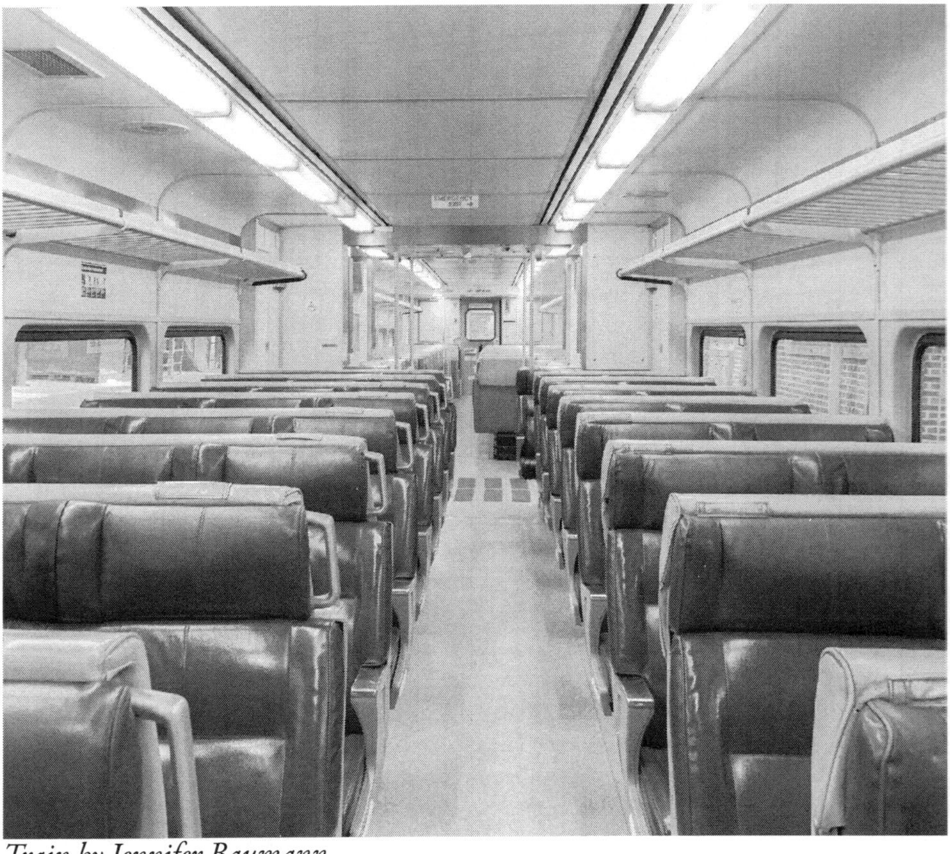

Train by Jennifer Baumann

Tom Burns

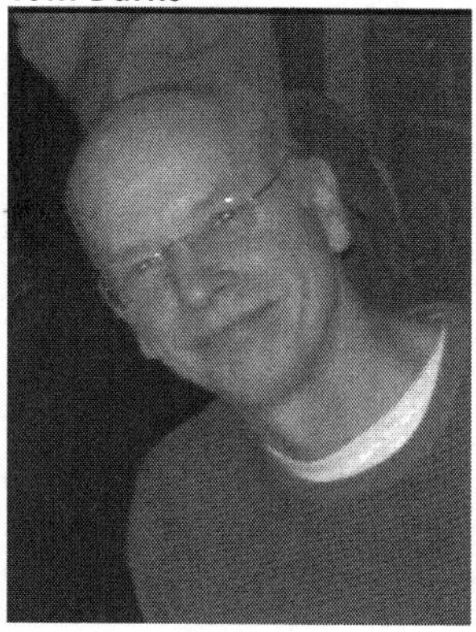

Way Up in the Parent-Filled Bleachers

MANY OF US WANTED TO HELP PATIENTS WHO SCREWED UP THEIR KIDS or to help the kids themselves but never did we expect to really mess up our own kids so much that they would need their own therapy—because we so wanted them to fill our own emptiness and resolve our sorrow with their exploits of the athletic, the academic, or the relational (even if) we only watched furtively and delighted secretly in the great job we did and how much we were the good parents they needed but had never experienced ourselves and then a therapist friend's teenager tells his therapist-parent to go fuck himself and another runs away on the Greyhound and another languishes, crying in loneliness unable to keep a boyfriend, rejecting anyone that likes her a lot, and so, freshly aware that our children are not immune from problems we seem to transmit from the past, I sat with my two daughters and my wife at the dinner table, mumbling that I needed to talk about a health matter or "issue" or something like that, and began to say "I have prostate—" getting hung-up on the "c" in "ca-cancer" and choked and finally got it out, even as I tried to hold back tears like Lou Gehrig or Ed Muskie, intent on mentioning all the good treatment options after which my eldest lowered her fork in slow motion from her mouth to her plate and set it down silently—or at least I heard no sound—as if in that moment her need for nourishment had been erased and she wiped away her tears and my wife tried to step in as I blubbered in the way that my mother blubbered when there was any calamity and I hated her for it and refused to talk but my wife, though distressed, managed to speak and my youngest daughter stoic as I

> "Many of us wanted to help patients who screwed up their kids or to help the kids themselves but never did we expect to really mess up our own kids so much that they would need their own therapy..."

had been forty years ago though I didn't fully trust that was her whole response, nor had it been mine—both she and her big sister asked good questions and interspersed with laughter we finally carried on with dinner, whole wheat pasta and some tomato spinach thing, the most uncarcinogenic meal we could ingest short of raw broccoli and bran buds, and anyway, it was a relief to be done with my disclosure, but then I started into another part—I couldn't seem to help myself—that was clearly for me and only me, saying that we hadn't wanted to burden them but my oldest said maybe too quickly that she was glad we told them and sadly, I saw my daughter attending me in the same way I'd attended my mother, but then convinced myself that it was a reflection of my daughter's maturity and empathy and filled with pride I could give her a standing ovation from way up in the parent-filled bleachers and then it fell to the youngest to ask the obvious but frightening question about whether or not the cancer would return and I told her that it almost never did, which was the truth though in part I wanted her to worry that it would and then I could milk the drama further for more attention, excitement, and sympathy, but near the end of the conversation—in a stab at grabbing even more by way of a sly and self-serving suggestion—I said, "so if somebody comes up to you and asks about your dad having cancer, be sure to tell them it's the slow-growing kind" and my oldest scoffed at this awkward reply and it hit me that she was right, that she was not I and that she would not dismiss her own reality in the service of her father's flight from his. Thank God.

This article is reprinted from Voices, Spring 2007. *The illness described is unrelated to what afflicted Tom last year leading to his death, but we find it uncannily apt as his final contribution to Voices. We wanted Tom's own voice to be part of this issue.*—Eds.

Lisa Zimmerman

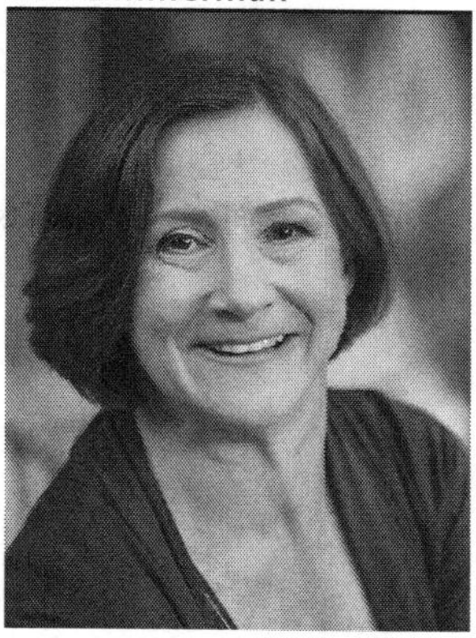

LISA ZIMMERMAN, MSW, is a psychotherapist and writer living and practicing in the Washington, D.C. suburbs. Her work has appeared in ROOM: A Sketchbook of Analytic Action and Kaleidoscope: Exploring the Experience of Disability through Literature and the Fine Arts. She is currently a student in the New Directions in Writing program through the Washington-Baltimore Center for Psychoanalysis.

Articles

Out of Bounds

I HAVE ALWAYS LOVED RULES. Where other people see confinement and constraint, I find clarity. Knowing what is allowed and what is considered forbidden provides me with its own sort of liberation. If I know what the bounds are, I can allow myself to expand without the fear of taking up too much space. Over the years, I have counted calories, aimed for 10,000 daily steps, and tracked my sleep cycles. Having targets to hit and limits not to exceed has brought me a singular comfort.

Being introduced to psychoanalytic psychotherapy in 2001 as a newly minted MSW opened a world surprisingly suited to my disposition. As a graduate student, I gravitated to cognitive behavioral therapy, with its crisp lists of cognitive distortions and its uniform battery of homework assignments. Negative feelings were born of incorrect thoughts; identify those thoughts and the feelings would resolve. Simple equations deliver guaranteed outcomes; suffering could be sorted into tidy boxes and taken away.

That confidence quickly eroded as soon as I met Javier, my first client at the HIV clinic where I worked after graduation. He had just been discharged from an inpatient hospitalization following a suicide attempt. The worst of his depressive symptoms had stabilized with medication, but a low-grade hopelessness persisted. Added to that was a skin picking disorder, making him too self-conscious to leave his apartment, much less socialize or look for work. His mother, a devout Catholic, made an anemic attempt to tolerate his sexuality but was never able to provide him the acceptance he craved. He longed to share his HIV diagnosis with her, but couldn't bear risking what little connection they maintained.

I was overtaken by the depth of his loneliness. I felt desperate to reach across the gulf between us, to provide some sort of balm. I tried frantically to recall some exercise or technique from my textbooks that I could offer in response, but the words that came out of my mouth sounded robotic. I suddenly felt like the foolish one, having ever believed that correcting negative thinking would be enough to address such despair - or even that negative thinking was something one could correct at all.

"What about his childhood?" asked my supervisor, instead of the direct guidance I'd hoped she'd give me. Disappointed as I was, it didn't come as a surprise. While I was immersed in learning CBT, my closest graduate school friends were studying psychodynamic theory. We spent many a lunchtime debating whether or not there was an unconscious and what purpose there was in dwelling on the past. They saw my approach as a superficial band aid; I saw theirs as overly subjective. But my paralysis with Javier seemed to give me no choice but to wonder whether there wasn't more to the psyche than met the eye.

As it turns out, there was much to explore in Javier's childhood. He was born to a single, working-class mother outside the capital of El Salvador. With hopes of finding economic stability, his mother left for the US when Javier was six. The understanding they had was that she would emigrate first and send for him once she had built a solid foundation. Javier stayed behind with his grandmother, surrounded by aunts, uncles, and a bevy of cousins.

Though never without people nearby, Javier was lonely. Sensitive and reserved from the outset, he felt his mother's absence profoundly. He was bullied in school and then sexually abused by an older cousin, all of which he endured in silence. His mother finally sent for him when he turned 17. Coming to the US provided an escape, yet he arrived to find a mother he felt he didn't know. Once again, he felt alone, navigating a new culture as well as his awakening sexuality.

It wasn't long into my work with Javier that I started borrowing my supervisor's texts on psychodynamic theory. I realized that his complex history, as well as many others that filled my caseload, could not be reduced to simple equations on worksheets. How could we analyze their thinking if they couldn't put words to, or even remember, their experiences? Studying Freud and his followers gave me a rich new perspective, one that felt much better suited to the task I faced. I began to see myself less of a mechanic responsible for fixing my clients' emotional distress and more of an archeologist who sought to unearth its roots.

Stimulated in ways I'd never been in graduate school, I was hungry to learn as much as I could. I enrolled that fall in a two-year certificate program in psychodynamic psychotherapy. It was 2003 and ego psychology and object relations dominated the curriculum. I soaked up the discussions around defenses and the unconscious. Thinking about projective identification and transference, splitting and countertransference, made my work, if not easier, far more meaningful.

What I hadn't anticipated was psychodynamic practice would provide me with a new set of rules to follow, a way to assess whether or not I was doing "good therapy." Although no instructor said anything this explicit, there were clear bounds we were to remain in if we were to call ourselves psychoanalytic psychotherapists. The Relational Turn ushered in by Stephen Mitchell (1988) was still in its adolescence and therapeutic neutrality was still the expectation. An early supervisor chided me for making small

"We need to remember across generations that
there is as much to learn as there is to teach."
—Gloria Steinem

talk with a client while escorting him to my office from the lobby downstairs. I became skilled in dodging questions about my vacations, certain that any answer would disrupt the transference.

There was another benefit to this way of working, a benefit that I didn't realize I'd needed. The imperative to be anonymous and opaque felt like a weight had been taken off my shoulders. If my presence was simply to be a blank screen for my clients' projections, I could let go of my worry about how the real me—the physical me—was perceived.

I was diagnosed with cerebral palsy at the age of two, after having been born with the umbilical cord wrapped around my neck and depriving my brain of oxygen. I wasn't yet walking when the doctors made the diagnosis and at that point it was uncertain how profound my disability would be. By the time I entered grade school, it was clear that the impact was relatively mild. Because balance and coordination remained a challenge, I never learned to ride a bike and I avoided anything else athletic. I attended therapy for a slight speech impediment that was fortunately often mistaken for a southern accent. Otherwise, though, my CP seemed to fade into the background. Being the pre-ADA 1970's, disability accommodations were rarely discussed in mainstream schools. If there was something I couldn't do, I learned to devise creative workarounds. Flying under the radar was what mattered most.

And flying under the radar became instinctive. I learned not to carry hot coffee across a crowded café, in the event that my tremor caused it to spill. I sat in the front of classrooms to avoid walking past my peers, putting my unsteady gait on display. I avoided public speaking to the extent that I could and went out of my way, in general, to avoid the spotlight.

"So, what do you have?" blurted a client during my first case management internship.

His question took me aback, but it did not come as a surprise. A part of me knew this moment would come; it always did. Though my CP lived on the periphery of my daily life and relationships, inevitably some curious acquaintance would need an explanation for my physical peculiarities. I knew intellectually that these inquiries were benign, but they always felt like a punch in the gut. It was as if I had failed in my efforts to camouflage my defects, and had lost my chance to be seen as an equal. I can't recall how I answered that client, but I know it involved choking back tears.

Moments like this notwithstanding, few of my clients seemed to be distracted by my physical differences—and those that were were either too polite or too embarrassed to ask. The limited extent of my impairment, together with the analytic mandate to

It was as if psychoanalytic theory provided me with a magical cloak. I was attuned, of course, to clients' transference and was not naive enough to pretend that my disability did not factor into that.

minimize my presence in the room, usually relieved the worst of my self-consciousness. It was as if psychoanalytic theory provided me with a magical cloak. I was attuned, of course, to clients' transference and was not naive enough to pretend that my disability did not factor into that. However, there was something freeing in believing that any discomfort someone felt about my body could be understood as projection. Any negative judgement a client harbored said more about them then it did about me. This was more than protection, this was power.

As the years passed, I fell into a comfortable rhythm in my work. My fears that my cerebral palsy would be an impediment to my therapeutic career faded. I was fortunate to see clients for years and do, what my analytic supervisors considered, "good therapy." In a handful of instances, my disability was addressed, but only when it was glaringly necessary. By and large, the fact that I was considered disabled rarely crossed my mind.

"I already told her that you have CP." My colleague, retiring in a month and eager to refer out his caseload, announced as he trailed me down the hallway. Boom. There it was. It always caught up with me, no matter how much I thought that it had receded from view.

I knew the client he was speaking of before he ever mentioned her name. I had seen Astrid around the clinic before, her deliberate, scissored gait hard to miss, even in the chaos of the waiting room. She rarely looked up from behind her overgrown bangs. I imagined she knew that she was being stared at. Now it was my turn to be the polite one. Despite a curious pull to watch her labor up the stairs, I always turned away.

Our first session filled me with unexpected anxiety. I knew that if I didn't address our shared condition out of the gate, it might feel like I was sweeping it under the rug, perhaps communicating that I saw it as a source of shame. But suddenly I was hit by a wave of a different sort of self-consciousness: what if I'm not disabled enough? Was she expecting a therapist whose body mirrored hers?

She told me that she was glad, if not surprised, to be referred to a therapist with CP. "For once, I won't have to explain myself," she offered with little elaboration—and I chose not to prod so early in our work. I assumed that she was referring to the sense of feeling defective, not to mention all the projections that the disabled must navigate. But I could only imagine that there is much she will have to explain. She does not have the privilege, I hastily presumed, of relegating her disability to the sidelines, as I do.

I was surprised to learn that Astrid's struggles with her disability did not dominate our sessions. She talked about relationship issues, frustrations at work, annoyances with family, similar to most of my other clients. Her depression was not, as her previous therapist stated in his notes, "due to her affliction." Instead, her deepest despair was about the political climate, especially as a queer woman whose rights were again under threat.

Her cerebral palsy, however, was not without its emotional impact. The pressure she felt at work was underscored by her belief that she must prove herself to be as competent as non-disabled colleagues. She had hobbies and a circle of friends, but at times resented the limitations her disability creates. She had learned that asking for help always carries a risk. Better to forgo opportunities than be singled out as a burden. I, of course, had no problem relating.

Months into our work together, I decided to go out on a limb, one that I knew would not be sanctioned by my former supervisors. I began, very tentatively, to sprinkle in self-disclosure to those sessions where she alluded to her cerebral palsy. I commiserated about the drudgery of physical therapy. I empathized when she spoke of her family's well-intentioned urgings to pull herself up by her bootstraps and downplay her needs. We laughed together when I shared my mother's frequent references to Helen Keller, both knowing that she is held up as the patron saint for so many disabled children.

To my relief, my opening up about pieces of my history did not have the catastrophic consequences that I'd feared. My occasional personal anecdotes did not open a Pandora's box of disclosure that destroyed the therapeutic boundaries. Nor was it some groundbreaking intervention that cured her depression. Counterintuitively, I believe that overtly bringing my CP into our work allowed me to see her as so much more than hers.

As I continued seeing Astrid, I began to notice a shift in my work with other clients, one that was at once subtle and profound. The vigilance, both about my physical difference and about being a "good therapist," started to ease. I no longer panicked when a client asked me where I was going on vacation; in some cases, I answered directly and in others I explored the inquiry. The rules that I had held as sacred began to feel somewhat arbitrary. I began to experiment with greater openness with other clients, starting to trust my own instinct and discretion. More importantly, perhaps, I started to trust in my relationships with clients. Time and time again, if there was progress in the treatment, it was seldom the result of some sophisticated interpretation I'd made. Instead, it arose from a co-created intimacy, one that allowed for my missteps and improvisation.

Recently, I was in session with a client whom I've seen for the better part of a decade. Although she is able-bodied, she has expressed affinity with the disability community, largely because of her ADHD and bipolar disorder. I'd signaled, through references to disabled authors, that I shared this affinity, but had never named my cerebral palsy explicitly. Without trepidation, I asked her whether she knew I had CP. She nodded enthusiastically, making it clear that I had stated the obvious. "It's been great," she continued. "You bring such a nuanced perspective. I see that things aren't so black and white and maybe I'm not broken."

I laughed inwardly, finally realizing that it was only when I let go of my beloved rules and analytic neutrality that healing could happen—both for my clients and myself. I put my magical cloak in the closet and breathed a deep sigh of relief

References:

Mitchell, S. (1988). *Relational Concepts in Psychoanalysis: An Integration.* Harvard University Press.

Commentary

I LOVE THIS AUTHOR'S PROFESSIONAL JOURNEY. I love that they allowed it to be shaped by patients, and that those patients took them all the way from the least relational to the most relational end of the field. And I get it. The personal and professional details are different of course, but every post-graduate training I've ever done has been an ode to a particular patient—someone I wasn't doing right by with the tools I had, someone I wanted to reach in a different way, someone who helped me grow.

Inspired by Javier, the author's first clinical transition is quite dramatic in its "and now for something completely different" quality. Do CBT and traditional psychoanalysis even belong in the same sentence? This transition was a conscious choice. It required going back to school to study the human psyche in a totally different way. Javier needed to be known from the inside out, like no one had ever known him before, and the author learned a whole new language in order to do so. It was still a one-person psychology, with lots of space for the therapist to hide out, but therapy got so much bigger and vastly more complex.

Coming out from behind the blank screen—or taking off the magical cloak—to be with Astrid in a different way required something else. Like the author, I've come to understand that transformational psychotherapy requires the therapist to have more skin in the game than anyone ever bargains for when they enter the helping profession. But I had so many teachers, supervisors, and theorists pointing the way. "Come on in, the water's fine!" they beckoned. With no help from Stephen Mitchell or anyone else, this author went rogue! And in this case the question wasn't "should I disclose what kind of music I like?" It was one that connected them to lifelong shame. That's courage.

At the same time, I imagine the author didn't have much of a choice. A deeply personal part of them was pressing to enter the conversation and eventually it spoke. Astrid responded in kind, and, sentence by sentence, they co-created the kind of intimacy that deep transformation both enables and requires. It's relational magic. That they then found their other therapeutic relationships deepening comes as no surprise. Anyone who brings all of who they are to the consulting room knows that growth is all about risk, all about going out of bounds, and that things are never the same. Thank you for articulating it so beautifully, Author.

—Stephanie Spalding

Svetlana Kreimer

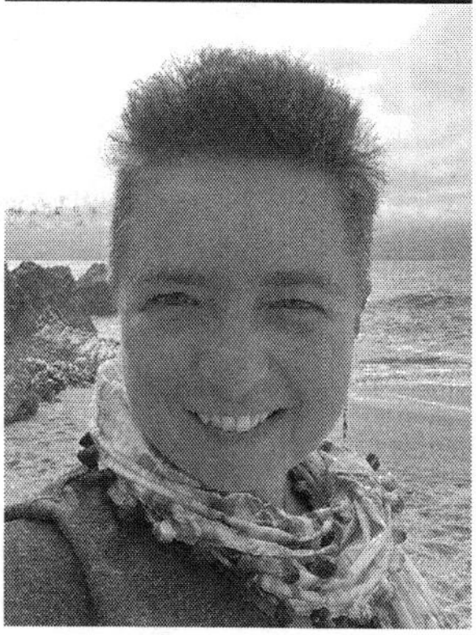

Svetlana Kreimer, LMFT works with diverse Silicon Valley families, couples and individuals, inviting growth through self-awareness, creative expression, and genuine human connection. As a Clinical Director at the Process Therapy Institute, she also supervises and trains budding therapists to discover their own voices amidst the confusion, grief and joy of their new clinical encounters. *sv.kreimer@gmail.com*

The Therapy of Allowance, or Master's Degree in Anything

Ask Master Don-or-NonDon if you have an important question about life, liberty, or the pursuit of anything. He is convinced he knows quite a bit. He even purchased a master's degree in "Anything." (By Don Hadlock, LMFT, from old Process Therapy Institute website)

"What, you don't know all fifteen stages of differentiation off the top of your head?", he asks, deadpan.

I, a trainee on the second week of a supervision group, freeze, desperately searching through all the lists and categories I learned during the last two years of schooling... and then see mischief in his eyes and flood with relief: He is joking. Wait, can you joke about these things?!

Don Hadlock, my mentor at the Process Therapy Institute, together with his life and work partner Carol Hadlock, was undoubtedly the best thing that happened to me as a therapist.

For many years of my work and studying in America I felt I never quite fit in—too quick to respond, too darkly humorous, too argumentative... It is only when I started working and training with Don and Carol in my clinical practicum 19 years ago that I was finally able to relax, learning to embrace all parts of myself... What a relief it was to have my Russian-Jewish cultural and personal quirks not just tolerated, but truly welcomed and even appreciated!

In addition to supervision, a weekly "mirror training" was an unusual, intensive experience. A trainee therapist would be observed in a session through a one-way mirror, and a supportive, experienced trainer would offer feedback in real time through an earpiece. I still remember many of these sessions vividly, as if they'd happened last week.

In one memory, with Don observing, the client talks about a string of bad decisions in her youth that led to a series of "rotten" and abusive relationships. She talks about letting go, forgiving those men, whom she sees now clearly as broken and abused themselves... To me, she appears collected and well-integrated, even tough, and I am impressed and pleased with her generosity.

Suddenly, Don's voice is in my ear: "Has she forgiven herself?" While not sure where that is coming from, I nonetheless repeat the question out loud.

Instantly, the client is quiet, pensive. Then she starts crying. Don's question unlocks the grief and self-loathing that were waiting all these years to be processed and understood. She connects with the young woman she had been, desperate, but also determined and strong, who did what she needed to do to persevere and escape the nightmare, thus leaving the past behind. The client is finally able to feel compassion for that confused and lonely, and so brave girl. Regrets and shame subside, no longer required to keep her moving. In my memory, at the end of the session I see a glimpse of what's possible—a woman, finally at peace.

I, however, remember feeling completely bewildered: How did Don know what to ask? She didn't bring up self-forgiveness, yet he sensed it was the missing piece...

Now, I look at my confused and frustrated past self with smile and compassion. It would take me many more years to accept that Don didn't have to know, but instead he would trust his experience and inquisitive intuition to guide his shot in the dark... and then deal with whatever transpired—whether profound release, or client's frustration, or no response at all.

Today, it is still Don's voice I hear when I tell my supervisees: "I have some news for you. The good one: You cannot do it wrong—it is the client who decides how to use your intervention in the moment, and you—staying present and intentional—will follow them and work with whatever reaction comes up. Unfortunately, it means there is also bad news: You cannot do it right either. It is still up to the client to decide how they choose to work."

And as I see the relief on my budding therapists' faces – my favorite supervision moment every time—I think: "Thank you Don, once again, for this gift."

—Master Don-or-NonDon,
Why do fools fall in love?
Signed, Unknown

—Dear Unknown,
Fools fall into everything. They fall into holes, into trouble, into merriment, as well as into love. The dictionary definition of fool is one who does not know he is not watching where he is going. The good news is, if enough fools fall into something, it will soon fill it up so there will be no risk of us falling into it. Hoping to meet you at the bottom of the heap,
Master Don-or-NonDon

Don loved making sense of the workings of the world. Partial to experiential in-the-moment work, with his engineering mind, he was always making sense of the inner mechanics of therapy, consciousness and growth. Looking for common unfolding processes with various humanistic approaches such as Gestalt or psychodrama, he translated it all into flowcharts as brilliant as they were visually flamboyant.

Being greatly influenced by Eastern spiritual philosophies he would make countless charts and teachings about "releasing attachments, being in the moment, connecting to Source..." With his white beard and kind round face, I often imagined him as a "Buddhist Santa Claus." He believed that the only way to invite our clients to release suffering and let go, would be for ourselves first to come from a place of ease and well-being.

While inspiring, this challenge also made studying with Don quite frustrating at times. "Just release resistance, people," he would say, "release resistance! Allow what is—remember, all is well..." He made it look easy, too easy. "Whether or not it is clear to you, the universe is unfolding as it should..." I didn't then recognize the quote from Desiderata poem (Max Ehrmann, 1927), and would feel my frustration rising: How can I "just release" my pain, my tension, my worry... Is he "bypassing"? Is he really that enlightened? How do I get there?

What was not clear to me then is that there is no "getting" or "staying" there, only patiently returning to that state of allowance and acceptance; catching myself slipping into countertransference and coming back anew with more awareness, over and over, often without a client's even noticing...

Thankfully, he didn't just preach, he showed us how to get there, into the therapeutic openness and connection of "I am ok, you are ok"; compassionate curiosity, creativity, both daring and tender playfulness... "Into the eye of the storm", into the pain and darkness we were invited to go with our clients again and again, to transcend and emerge on the other side with a larger sense of self and a wider perspective of ownership, liberation and healing. And all that with a good dose of gentle humor on the side.

—Master Don-or-NonDon,
Is there a way to connect to the source, that profound silent stillness out of which all springs?
Signed, Tim

—Dear Tim,
Some people try to sneak up on it so as not to disturb the stillness, but alas this does not work. Others try to search for the spigot with which to make the connection, but alas this leads only to eye fatigue. Some clean house and release all the junk that is covering it, only to discover that the connection is already there.
One who needs to keep cleaning,
Master Don-or-NonDon

Some people preferred Carol's down-to-earth, straightforward kindness—a safe relief from Don's daring style. I loved them both; still, as he tried to teach courage to all of us, I remember at times resisting his fearless challenge, preferring to experiment with safety and creativity at my own pace.

In another mirror session, processing a dream where the client was trying to run away from a hideous monster that kept pursuing her, I suggested she "redream" and complete it in the "here-and-now." Together we started running from the monster, brainstorming more ways to hide in the imaginary scene.

In my memory, I am hearing Don in my earpiece: "Let's face the monster. Tell her to stop and look back. Let's confront him." Again and again, I choose to ignore him, and again and again the monster catches up with my client. She is scared; perhaps so am I, for I don't want to follow Don's suggestion. Isn't my job to help the client be safe, to protect her? Yet there is no safety from her monster in the dreamland she describes – no matter where we hide, there he is.

I am hearing impatience creeping up in Don's voice; he really wants me to be brave. The dream is stuck in the loop. Finally, I give in: "Stop. Turn back and look at him. Tell me what you notice."

The client agrees. She gasps. She reports a terrible burning smell… She has an insight, a memory from 9/11 in New York, where she was that day. Feelings are coming to the surface; a chance is here to work with the trauma that the monster represents…Our time is up. A sense of disappointment at the missed opportunity is burned into my memory.

During the debriefing, while Don was not thrilled with me, he was supportive: Nothing is a mistake, I did what I could when I was ready for it. A valuable lesson is learned—I don't want to wait till the end of the session for a permission to face my fears—a golden opportunity might lie there. My own students, terrified to make a wrong "unsafe" move, will be hearing this story in years to come.

At the same time, while working hard to embolden us, Don consistently invited us to pause and stay still, to get out of the client's way of processing, to be "a lazy therapist… a placebo for the client to use as they need…" "Your first job is to shine your light, to be present. Your Being is more important than your Doing."

And so I learned to sit with discomfort, with grief, with my helplessness to "fix," to change anyone but myself, with existential limitations of being in a world full of suffering… and to trust that with all that, I am enough. To trust that perhaps my bold presence is a worthy enough offering on our collective quest for peace, just one person at a time – even with my own dark places, passionate nonconformity, twisted Russian jokes and all. For a girl raised in an atheistic, godless Soviet Union—if there is any spiritual spark in my practice and in my relationship with the universe, it is also Don's gift to me.

—Master Don-or-NonDon,
Where can I get a degree in humor therapy?
Signed, Wondering

—Dear Wondering,
Your question is certainly a laughing matter. You must get the recommendation of 4 people who have said your humor has improved the quality of their life, see the joyful absurdity of the world, and stop taking yourself so seriously. When this is complete, send a registered letter to yourself issuing yourself a degree in humor therapy. Ridiculously yours,
Master Don-or-NonDon

Perhaps my most memorable experience happened during the supervision where Don was teaching us to work with suicidal ideation. It is a sad and scary issue, and understandably, many of us were anxious as we approached it. Don, however, rooted in his spiritual and holistic beliefs, was not afraid of the thought of death, nor of inviting the dark subject into the work. He believed that some parts need to die in order to transcend and re-integrate—"resurrect, re-birth"—and in order to make space for other processes to emerge.

So here he is in the group, so fresh in my mind, asking for a volunteer to demonstrate his use of guided imagery in exploring a wish of death and inviting it to completion. I raise my hand. Don tells me to visualize going ahead, following my wish to kill myself. Not a stranger to morbid ideation, I eagerly dive in. "Let me know when you're dead." I am there. "Notice your experience... what you are aware of... is there an image...? Feel how it is for you to see yourself there..." I become aware of a surprising and wonderful peacefulness that overtakes me. I am in a beautiful place, surrounded by sunlight; there is no pressure to do or be any different; no pain; no more responsibilities or regrets... As a matter of fact, it is quite blissful. Don lets me rest in this magical place, and after a while invites me back into my body, into the present, into the room. I feel great.

As I open my eyes, I see that all my groupmates are vigorously scribbling in their notepads, faces scrunched with concentration, so burdened with thoughts, so different from my experience! A thought comes: "Wow, I am glad that my death can be used in the service of learning for others. I guess my life is not wasted after all."

Immediately recognizing it as a pinnacle of my martyrdom and ridiculous self-sacrificial psychological programming, I start laughing. I am aware that to others I probably look hysterical; it is confirmed by the looks of horror I am now getting; but I just cannot stop, it is that funny. Finally, wiping my eyes from the tears of laughter, I am able to exhale and explain the reason for my amusement. It is a profound release and relief. "See," Don chimes in, "you didn't even have to kill yourself to feel better."

"You're never going to be whole while you have these physical bodies. You're connected—you are actually whole—but you can never really fully connect to wholeness with these bodies. ...I'm not sure if you heal when you die, either. You know, you just keep transcending. The whole idea of healing is a myth. It's the idea that something's wrong. There is nothing wrong."

After the practicum I left Don and PTI to explore some greener pastures, but later returned for more wisdom and fearlessness of the Process Model approach. I kept coming back, first as an intern, advancing my learning into Don's charts and techniques, later as a supervisor and trainer when he needed more people to assist in running the Institute.

All that teaching came useful in January 2020.

I often dreamed of working alongside Don, and got my wish in 2018 for a short couple of years. Little did I know that he would leave us abruptly and without a warning right before the COVID pandemic ("what a lucky escape", I sometimes can't help thinking). I like to believe that he went as joyously into the final transcendence, to his beloved Consciousness, as I did with his help into my restful imagery. With Carol's not working any more at the time, also passing away soon after, we, a few bewildered apprentices, were left to mind the shop without our dear teachers, who for 35 years willed and breathed the place into existence.

It felt like we were children running the house without adult supervision, pretending to be grown-ups in their parents' shoes and too baggy clothes. The pandemic added a surreal sense that "life will be completely different from now on, even more than you previously thought possible". Thankfully, we were also supported by Don's loyal business partner, PTI Executive Director at the time, Don Arnoldy. He stayed with us two years longer than planned, until our knees stopped wobbling.

Did we survive? Yes, we did, don't ask me how. I guess for me, I just felt an obligation and stubborn desire to see Don and Carol's work continued. I felt a responsibility to pass their vision on to new cohorts of students, so they too could learn to be still, and brave, and thoughtfully playful with human suffering and resilience.

To my not-quite-surprise and grateful relief, the Process Model held its own in translation to telehealth. While missing sandplay toys or Gestalt-type experientials with chairs and pillows in the room, the main principles of working in the moment, inviting introspection, deepening in a metaphor, and following processes to completion, still allowed clients to grieve, break through internal barriers, and accomplish whatever work they needed to do.

With time, with some older clinicians leaving to pursue their calling elsewhere while new generations of therapists keep joining us for training and supervision, I became the Clinical Director of the Process Therapy Institute, title once held by Don. I joke that instead of making a career, if you wait by the river long enough, all the ancient Clinical Directors would float by, and then the career will make you. So, for now I am it.

—Master Don-or-NonDon,
Why does my counselor just nod and grunt "Un-huh?"
Signed, Somewhat Frustrated

—Dear Somewhat,
Well, it's the way they have been trained. Most counselors go to the School of Hard Nods. The grunting is one way they keep themselves awake. Noddingly yours,
Master Don-or-NonDon

Don was never concerned with publishing or building fame; but after two years of simplifying and toning down his exuberant charts and collecting articles and quotes from his class recordings, we are finally about to publish a book on the Process Model – a tribute to his life's work. I look forward to a day when his writings will be accessible to the larger public, even if it is 30 years overdue.

I realized I was doing a good job of absorbing and passing on my mentors' wisdom when a supervisee from a different institution, not previously aware of Don and Carol's role in my life, shared her recent dream of an unusual supervision session with me:

"... In my dream I notice you looking beyond me at my background, and I see an expres-

sion of recognition across your face. Next, I see you walking down a spiral staircase towards me, and even more surprising, you are followed by two of your friends. One of them is an older white man with glasses. He has kind eyes and a warm smile. He explains to me that you all used to work together, but about three years ago you had to go your separate ways. But you are now working together again, and you are all so happy about it that the three of you decided to supervise me that day together."

Later she wrote about it in her final class paper:

"We spent some time working the dream, and before the end of our session my supervisor shared that she had two mentors. One of them was an older white man, who wore glasses. He passed away shortly before the COVID-19 pandemic, now just over three years ago. So for her, my dream was "as if" her mentor were still with her, guiding and supporting her and her work.

I was and continue to be quite moved by my supervisor's reverie of my dream, both for the positive impact it had on her and in helping me realize that as one of her supervisees, I am now also a member of her professional lineage."

And indeed, it is so. Sometimes, after a particularly lovely session, I come out of the office and notice a graceful white heron crossing a dusky-purple sunset sky. I believe then, that on the other side of that immense one-way mirror, Don is quite pleased with me.

—Dear Master Don-or-NonDon,
You say we must change alone, and need others so that we can change. Why do we need others for our change?
Grateful Universe Student

—Dear Grateful Universe Student,
We change alone to be discrete and because we are the only one who can truly dress ourselves anyway. Yet without seeing what others are wearing, how can we gauge what it is we want to change into. Here's watching you,
Master Don-or-NonDon

Commentary

In this rather magical account of the writer's development under the guidance of her mentors, we see her taking in their ways of being in the psychotherapy work. We psychotherapists are the instruments we use as we sit with those who come to us, and keeping our instrument tuned is our obligation as clinicians. This is a story of that tuning. What happens with her in supervision sessions allows her to be with patients in new ways. The bravery and the tenderness exemplified by both of her mentors gets internalized and carried forward by her. At the article's end, we see how powerful the transmission was in her own session as a supervisor when an uncanny dream occurs. A beautiful conclusion.

—Molly Donovan

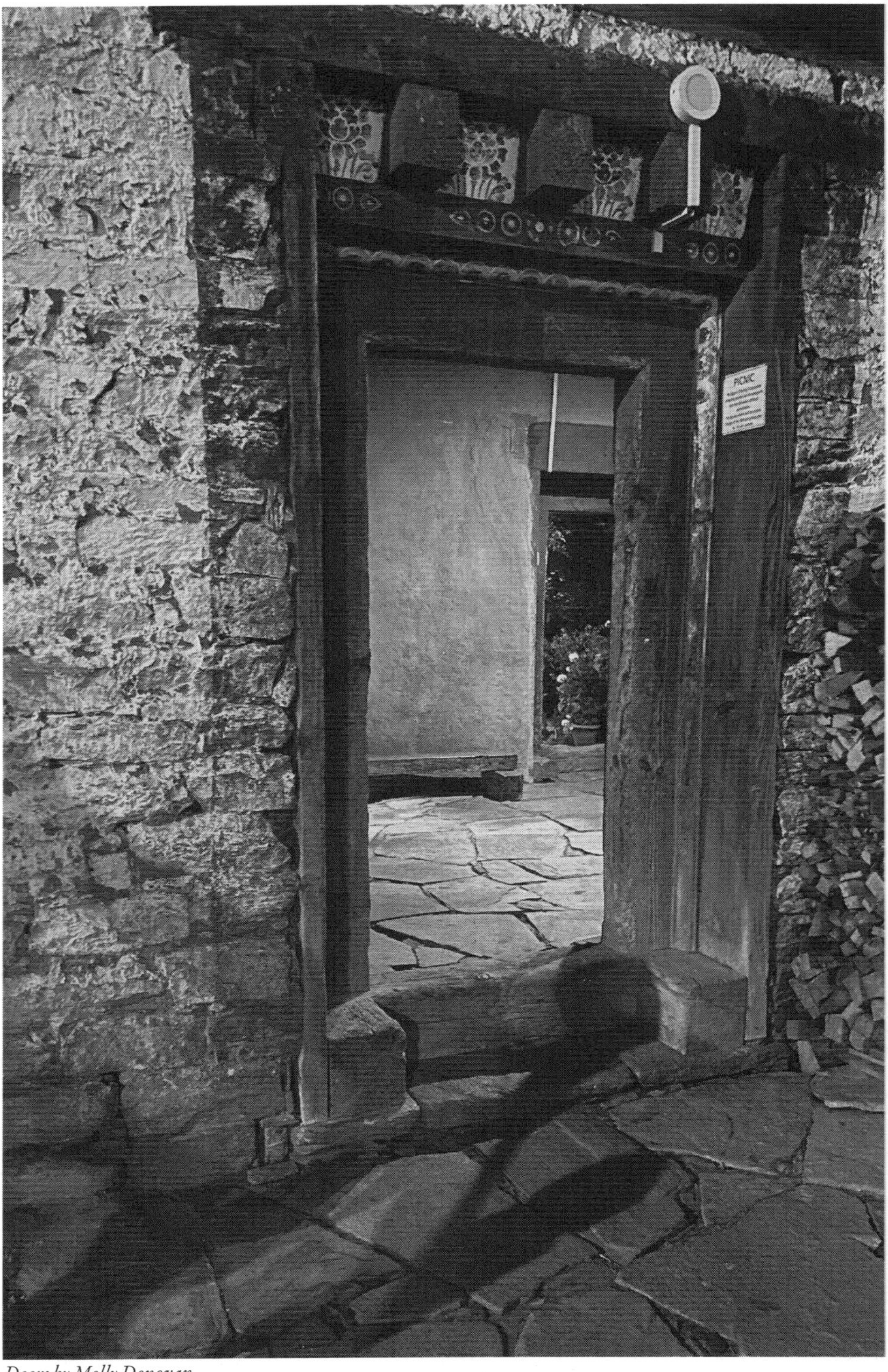

Doors by Molly Donovan

Doris Jackson

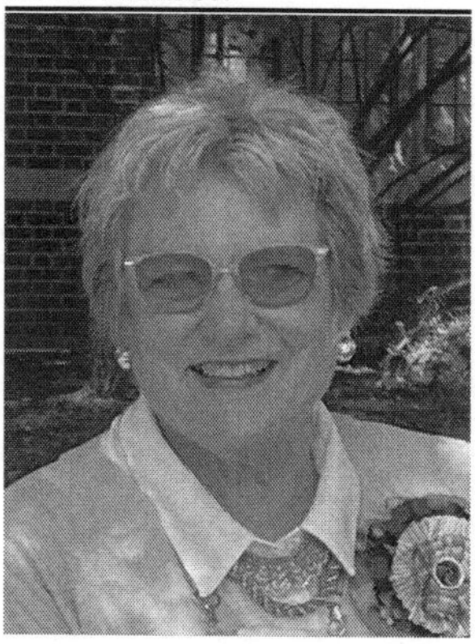

DORIS JACKSON PHD, is a Fellow of the Academy and former co-editor of Voices. She has presented multiple workshops at AAP meetings. In 2008 she and Lyn Sommer and Laurie Michaels created the AAP Scholarship program, and Doris has co-chaired the Scholarship committee since then. She has a private psychotherapy practice in Boston Massachusetts, treating individuals, groups and couples.
dorisj@comcast.net

What Do Young Therapists Want?

The editors of this issue of Voices had an idea: rather than telling our (to us) fascinating stories to the new generations, we should ask some younger members of our community what they want from us senior therapists. I was given the task of asking, and it was my pleasure to receive some answers.

What follows are five responses to the question "What do young people in AAP want from older members?" The answers are various—appreciative, complex, and challenging. To my mind, they add up to a description of good parenting, while modeling professional lives in progress.

It can be hard for us longtime AAP-ers to remember that we now occupy the position of the beloved (and sometimes feared) elders from our past. In days gone by we looked upon those elders as holding in their hands the gifts of recognition, wisdom and legitimacy. But us? Hey—we're just folks, right? Doing our best to do the work of the psychotherapist.

But—like it or not—we are the elders now. And elders, like parents, have no choice but to hold power, and be seen as the givers, or withholders, of caring and regard. We can give the gift of our time and our attention to the young, and this can make all the difference in our community. At the same time, we cannot avoid being seen as role models, for good or for ill. The way we meet the milestones of aging is being observed. And the way we engage with a challenge from younger members will accrue to our credit or our discredit.

A common theme in these responses is the wish to be seen, to be welcomed and claimed. The older members are invited, or in some cases thanked for giving at-

> "Of course, there is the wish to be mentored, to have the hard-won expertise of the veterans shared with up-and coming professionals."

tention and caring to newer members. In a memorable phrase, one person wrote of knowing there are some in AAP who "take delight in my growth." When the triumphs of the young are a delight to their elders, that is to me the essence of good parenting, in which the self can be put aside and subsumed in the other.

Of course, there is the wish to be mentored, to have the hard-won expertise of the veterans shared with up-and-coming professionals. Many in this community regularly do work to pass on what we have learned. But more powerful than any teaching is the I—Thou engagement that these newer AAP members report with older members. I loved that one writer asked to be accepted and cared for even while being awkward and whiny, and even while asking for too many wishes. Overall, these writers are eager for lively connection with the older generations, including in play, or in what one writer referred to as "laughter and vibrance. "

Some expressed the need for us to be role models, standing up for justice and inclusion and helping young therapists develop "fortitude" for the hard times we are living through. One writer said she wanted to find her clinical center, or "voice", even in the midst of chaos; and she told of witnessing her supervisor model this, including in AAP community meetings. In a passage I found moving, one writer appreciated our community for honoring the need for mourning, as we elders age, lose comrades and confront our own mortality.

On the shadow side is the challenge for us to see and respect newer members of AAP even when they are angry. One writer calls us to live up to the motto we in AAP often invoke—"more curiosity, less judgment." She asks us to hold space for the relationship between the generations even when it is contentious. Several writers wanted us to examine our own motives and to think critically about problems in our Academy and our world. Reading this I thought of songs of the 60's—urgent pleas for the older generation's support, even when the "new road" seems foreign. In my head I was singing Neil Young: "Old man take a look at my life, I'm a lot like you". I heard echoes of Dylan's words: "Come fathers and mothers, throughout the land. And don't criticize what you don't understand" and ... "Please get out of the new [road] if you can't lend your hand."

I have enjoyed being in communication with these young clinicians. Their courage and thoughtfulness in responding to this prompt bode well for our organization.

Fostering my Clinical Voice by Camilla Dorment

Camilla Dorment, LICSW, is a psychotherapist in Washington D.C. She practices in Dupont Circle where she treats individuals, couples, and groups. Camilla draws primarily on psychodynamic and existential theory, and believes that expressive treatments, like writing and art, can be central to healing. camilla@camilladorment.com

As a younger member of AAP I am confident that mentorship from older AAP members will foster my growth in one realm in particular: fine-tuning my clinical voice. Through countless community meetings and process groups, I have soaked up wisdom and insight from elder AAP members who have helped me improve my self-expression and clarify my goals as a psychotherapist. I have been given the grace, curiosity and room to explore my own boundaries—gifts for which I am so grateful. As I try to remain whole during turbulent seasons, my hope is that older AAP members will continue to share their experiences of finding their own clinical voice.

As a parent of a toddler, I often feel called upon to remain unflappable and sturdy in the face of chaos. There is a particular memory of my supervisor, Gary Frankel, a beloved older AAP member, reflecting those qualities for me. I had come to the session quite harried, with blood dripping down my left knee, having fallen off an electric scooter. After cleaning up the wounds with some bandaids, I was struck by how grounded Gary stayed in response to me. His ability to meet me with warmth and centeredness, and to help me observe how I can get in my own way—both figuratively and literally (!)—was a corrective emotional experience.

Those Who Delight in My Growth by Marvice Marcus

Marvice Marcus, PhD, is a licensed psychologist in North Carolina. Currently, Marvice divides his time between psychotherapy and overseeing a clinical training program. He is an avid reader, with interests ranging from psychoanalysis to cultural studies and critical social theory. marvice@interioritycc.com

Our world is changing. It is becoming increasingly difficult to experience and sustain wellness. Cultural and political unrest along with systemic inequality belie the most fundamental principles of our society. In choosing a "professional home" my intent was to invest in an organization that earnestly looks at its strengths and areas of growth when grappling with matters of identity, history, and human connection. While perfection eludes the Academy, I am confident that, within it, I can discuss significant matters with those who delight in my growth.

For me, "sitting at the feet of elders" is a demonstration of care and a cultural requisite that preserves wellbeing. Receiving mentorship and guidance from older members of the Academy creates a bridge between generations. To address the concerns that plague our society, critical conversations that include acknowledgment of wrongdoing, challenges to neutrality, and the transmission of diverse epistemologies are imperative.

"Receiving mentorship and guidance from older members of the Academy creates a bridge between generations."

Ideally, as a member of the Academy, I will engage with peers, new and old, who think critically and value self-reflection. I want to dialogue with members who are rigorous in their analyses of human behavior and emotional suffering. While culture and tradition promote belonging, I endeavor to associate with members who are also suspicious of belonging and thus know that culture is about conformity. At the same time, cultivating belonging ensures that individuals feel valued and included. Elders and senior members of the Academy share in the goal of creating a climate of acceptance and

> "At the same time, cultivating belonging ensures that individuals feel valued and included. Elders and senior members of the Academy share in the goal of creating a climate of acceptance and hospitality."

hospitality. When mentorship and belonging go hand in hand, they strengthen organizational cohesion, drive innovation, and support long-term success. With these factors, the pursuit of growing the therapist, in my mind, is even more worthwhile.

There are many kind and warm people who welcome me, each year, with genuine interest and open arms. Our interactions come with laughter and vibrance—we might even shed a tear or two. Hearing Gloria Beller regale the BIPOC group with words of wisdom and encouragement is a delight. Drs. Doris Jackson and Don Murphy held me with affection during my scholarship group, a container that was threatened by racial prejudice, among other biases. Years later, my experience of cofacilitating a group with Don was such a treat! Having Carrie Phillips scream my name in the middle of the lobby in Memphis was magical. Truly unmatched, Dr. Murray Scher's Fathers and Sons group was exceedingly special to me, as I was reminded that being fatherless does not mean I am alone. I can also appreciate a man whose fashion is almost as good as mine. Drs. Douglas Cohen, Penelope Norton, Fern Beu, and Gary Frankel are wonderful and softhearted faces to me. Dr. Jonas Horwitz is someone who will seize the moment in a group, willing to give and receive feedback, in a manner that is steady and appropriately humorous.

Finally, though closer to me in age, Sean LeSane, Tyler Beach, Renée Burwell, Liz Marsh, Michael Stahly, and Hayden Dawes have so much insight to offer new members. Experiencing their kindness and witnessing their navigation of the Academy has been invaluable to me.

Without question, these pleasant and constructive interactions became steppingstones toward membership for me. I am looking forward to more cross generation dialogues, more play, and the next time someone insists on having a "moment" with me before going into the restroom.

Developing Fortitude by Aaron Severn

Aaron Severn, LICSW, works with adults and couples in a private practice setting in Washington, DC. He began his involvement with AAP as an AAP scholar in 2023 before becoming an associate member last year. Prior to becoming a therapist, Aaron had a 15-year career working for a renewable energy trade association. He lives in DC with his spouse and two children. awsevern77@gmail.com

WHAT I WANT, AND MOST VALUE, FROM OLDER AAP MEMBERS, IS THEIR MENTORSHIP AND WISDOM. I think about David Pellegrini introducing me to the AAP community, which has become my professional "home", where I feel loved. I recall the deeper insight I developed while simultaneously experiencing and witnessing the care and skill of my early scholars' group leaders: Gloria Myers Beller, Steve Ingram and Doris Jackson. I reflect on Gordon Cohen taking time to meet with me as I become a more active AAP member.

As our nation descends into authoritarianism and my security feels threatened in a way I have never experienced, I find and want to hear more from older members by hearing about their extensive personal and professional experiences. Their collective wisdom during this uncertain time can be an invaluable resource for me as I work on developing fortitude to keep growing as a therapist and to continue caring for my community.

Inviting Curiosity by Hilary Hla

Hilary Hla, PsyD., is the Associate Director of Swarthmore College Counseling & Psychological Services (CAPS). They also run a small private practice and hold various roles in professional organizations including the Philadelphia Society for Psychoanalytic Psychology (PSPP) and the American Academy of Psychotherapists (AAP). Hilary stands in the spaces across multiple identities, as a genderqueer, queer and invisibly disabled multiracial Burmese-American. Outside of the therapy office, Hilary enjoys singing, cooking, swimming, indoor gardening, and connecting with loved ones, including their sweet orange tabby cat, Silvio. dr.hilaryhla@gmail.com

My 'wants' from older AAP members are twofold. One is already being met: I want to learn from older AAP members how to age and change and mourn and die with grace and wisdom. I appreciate the way AAP holds space for these milestones that often come later in life.

I've experienced my other want as more difficult to get. I wish for older AAP members to be curious about me, about their own reactions to me and my views, and about the distribution of power between us. I don't need other people to hold the same views as me in terms of sociopolitical ethos. Instead, the curiosity I wish for would ideally preserve space between us in such a way that I would not feel older members are standing in the way of my growth and actualization. In other words, please clear the path I am walking for me to become who I am meant to be, and don't stand in my way if you don't agree with me. I welcome challenges but would also want others to examine their challenge before launching it towards me.

> "I wish for older AAP members to be curious about me, about their own reactions to me and my views, and about the distribution of power between us."

Ideally, this would preserve space between us for us to connect and relate in ways that feel gratifying to both of us. It would allow interpersonal dynamics to emerge, instead of collapse as I sometimes feel they do at present, when my second request isn't honored. When I know someone does not consciously or unconsciously want to stand in the way of my actualization, it allows trust to develop. I know this because I have experienced it at AAP, with some elders. I feel hopeful that the AAP community is spacious enough for such curiosity to exist, and that we can foster relationships that contain disagreements as well as respect for one another's stage of development.

Daring to Want by Alec Addleton

Alexandra "Alec" Addleton Rigdon, MS, CET I, lives in Atlanta Georgia with her husband and baby son. A visual artist and experiential counselor-in-training, she finds joy in empowering others by maintaining reverence for their adaptability and creative spontaneity. She received an AAP scholarship award in 2023 and hopes to become a member soon. Insatiably curious and passionate, she offers those around her authenticity and empathy, often inspiring them to courageously express themselves in the safety of attuned connection. alecsart@gmail.com

I want older AAP members to grow in public with me.

I want older AAP members to model how to examine biases.

I want older AAP members to help me embody myself differently.

I want older AAP members to amplify, empower, and support disenfranchised voices.

I want older AAP members to show me how to care less about what others think about me.

I want older AAP members to demonstrate how to emote and process challenging experiences.

I want older AAP members to see and hear me accurately when I act or share with courageous authenticity.

I want older AAP members to share themselves with me, especially the parts they find most challenging to claim.

I want older AAP members to provide me with constructive feedback that may help me help myself and my clients better.

I want older AAP members to experiment with engaging with and moving through conflict and messiness personally and in relationship.

As someone with experience of not feeling allowed to want, I'm proud to have permitted my inner whiny baby to want so much of all of you. I hope you won't hold it against me and fear that some will. I also feel compelled to let you know that many of you already are and do these things exceptionally well. I'm eager to get to know you better and to share myself as clumsily as possible at every opportunity.

And gladly would he learn, and gladly teach.

—Geoffrey Chaucer

Penelope Norton

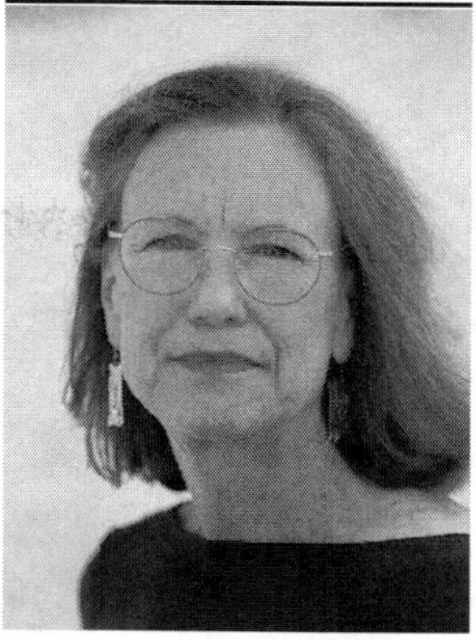

Penelope Norton, PhD practices psychotherapy with children, teens, adults and seniors in Ormond Beach, Florida. Like most senior therapists, she is unapologetically integrative and eclectic in her approaches to therapy. Most recently she incorporates experiences in the natural world into her work through Ecotherapy and Forest Bathing.

Becoming a Play Therapist

"To turn, turn, will be my delight, 'til by turning, turning, we come round right" —Shaker Hymn

As a child, I went out to play with my friend Eddie a few weeks after a tornado had destroyed his house and damaged mine. In our play, we hid from the tornado in a ditch, replicating his actual experience. We protected my dolls and his dog from the wind; we expressed our fear. He chose the play that day, and I intuited the need to go along with his lead. This may have been the first time I engaged in play therapy, but it was certainly not the last.

There is literature on the development of psychotherapists, positing that they grow toward the use of common factors in psychotherapy, regardless of therapeutic orientation. And that patients teach therapists to move from orthodox interventions toward more inclusive, fluid techniques appropriate to the client (Behan, 2022; Řiháček & Danelova, 2016; 2018; Thoma & Cicero, 2009). The work of Jean Piaget (1975) described cognitive development as a continual process of assimilation and accommodation, integrating new material into an existing framework until the creation of a new framework. And particularly in the development of women, it is difficult to determine which changes are due to the social context in which they live and which changes unfold from some inner, innate growth trajectory.

The story of my development as a therapist for children exemplifies this combination of assimilation and accommodation, toward increasing use of common factors in psychotherapy, and the zeitgeist of thought regarding play therapy as it evolved over the 50-years in

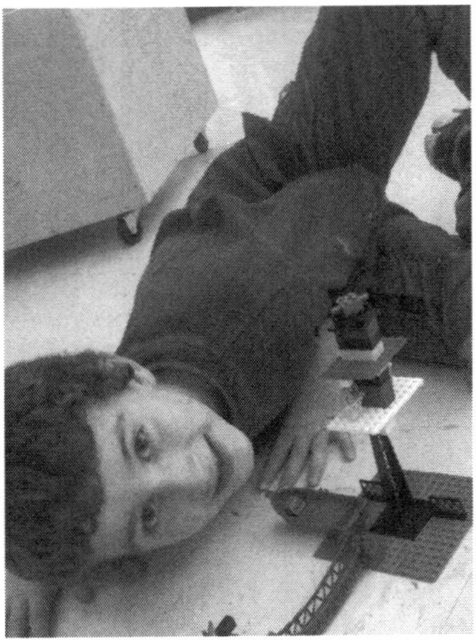

which I have practiced. Accordingly, this account toggles between the evolution of play therapy as it has shifted over time, and my own development as a child therapist. It is impossible to separate whom I have become from the external influences on me, including theorists, supervisors, and experiences in the playroom, or from some inborn and intrinsic growth.

Most children I see in play therapy have, like Eddie, experienced trauma. I have seen children traumatized by abuse, by storms, by fires, by animal attacks, by traumatic losses of family members, by car accidents, and by gunshot wounds. These traumas presented themselves repeatedly in my office, with innumerable "you can't make this up" occurrences that leave behind a hurt child. Literature and training prepared me poorly for this, as post-traumatic stress disorder (PTSD) was not a diagnosis given to children when I began my work. Despite diligent and thorough reading, the psychotherapy literature offered me only technique and theory that obscured underlying trauma. Yet, when I am at a loss, I look with curiosity to supervisors and to literature for guidance.

When I began studying psychology related to children, Freud predominated. After the publication of Freud's *Little Hans* (1909), there have been more than a 100-years of descriptions of alleviating children's trauma related distress through psychotherapy. Freud heavily interpreted Hans' trauma, which Freud attributed to Hans' oedipal conflicts. Interpretation was the active intervention in this framework. But I believed that the death of the horse was the actual trauma to be addressed, not some sort of screen memory. This conflict between treatment, interpretation, and theory first became clinically relevant to me during graduate school. I began treating a 14-year-old in the inner-city clinic during my practicum. She was very distressed, crying, and anxious when I began seeing her. She disclosed that her uncle, the owner of an ice cream store in her neighborhood, had sexually assaulted her. When I presented this case in group supervision, my very senior powerful male supervisor became focused on her oedipal sexual desires for her uncle. My fellow students remained glued silently to their seats while I silently wrestled with conflict between my own understanding of my patient and my distress over what had occurred to my client, and then, my distress over the supervisor's view. This did not sit well with me.

During the 1920s and 1930s, therapists such as Anna Freud, Frieda Fromm Reichman, Melanie Klein and Margaret Lowenfeld advanced treatment for children in the use of play as children's language of free association and emotion. In their methods, a therapist could function as a kind of second mother figure to a young client with internalizing symptoms. Instead of interpreting children's play, therapists became facilitators of *unrestricted* play. For example, Fromm Reichman is said to have allowed a child to smear feces on her in unrestricted permissive play. On the one hand, these pioneers embraced maternal transference from the child, and on the other, Fromm Reichman, surprisingly, coined the expression schizophrenogenic mother, a misogynistic and *mother blaming* view of women whose children were psychotic.

I also worked within this model with children, utilizing as techniques both unrestricted play and children's attachment to me as a mother figure. In my view this model had two significant faults. One, the mess in the playroom took forever to clean, generating negative countertransference about the work involved in clean-up of clay, sand, water, and countless toys. The second challenge had to do with confusion, for the child patient and for me, about mothering. If I attached to the child in a motherly way, (which due to my make-up was all too easy) it blinded me to some of the child's communications. In one such situation, when a child was showing me anger, and I persisted in my motherly ways exactly as if the child was still affectionate, my supervisor asked about this motherly countertransference. She said, taking a drag on her cigarette, "For God's sakes, you can sublimate that!"

In my opinion, these approaches involving the child's attachment to the therapist as a mother, colluded with a profession that held negative views about the role of mothers in a troubled child's life. To me, my motherly attachment ran the risk of "splitting" between me and the child's mother. Splitting occurred all the more easily given children's concrete, black and white thinking in which one mother could be "good" while the other "bad." How could I hinder easy collaboration with the child's mother by cementing mother-blaming, which eroded my own sense of self as a woman?

During the 1940s Virginia Axline's (1947; 1974) version of play therapy, aligned play therapy with Carl Rogers' person centered therapy (Rogers, 1951). Both Axline and Rogers had a more respectful, collaborative approach with parents and with mothers of their patients. While working with their ideas I had a motherly supervisor, who in her nonprofessional life was the mother of three children. She was the first psychologist involved in my training to express interest in and curiosity about my parents as people. One day, while complaining about a mother who felt she could no longer bring her child (my patient) to therapy, my supervisor broke her own non-directive and motherly protocol and simply told me what to do: "Call that mother, be gracious, tell her you understand her stresses, and let her know that your door will be open if anything changes". I did. Three months later, they returned to the clinic and my work helping the child resumed.

As I grew in my ability to manage my countertransference, I discarded interpretation as a technique with children and collaborated better with parents. I still sought solutions to the shadow side of unrestricted play and the nuances of my relationship with my child clients. Some answers to these dilemmas emerged through the contributions to play therapy of Haim Ginott, and D.W. Winnicott.

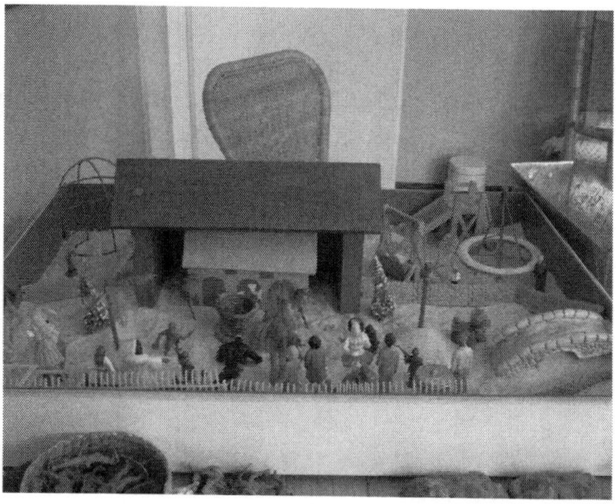

Ginott was concerned with the management of anger and the development of character of the child. This was his attempt to facilitate children's strength of character, and he wrote: "In adults, character determines experience; in children, experience determines character" (Ginott, 1968, p. 43).

Ginott's (1961) gentle techniques for setting limits within the session, and his non-directive language limited damage to the therapeutic relationship while in the playroom. My ability to set limits protected the healing experience of the child in therapy (i.e., I protected the therapeutic frame). This enabled me to no longer fear a massive clean up after the session or an angry countertransference to a child who might be messy. Utilizing Ginott's language helped me protect each child's experience while in the playroom with me. Experience was the healing focus rather than interpretation, unrestricted play, or maternal transference. For example, Ginott believed that therapists should not ask questions of children, a wisdom that was hard for me to learn as a therapist. But children receive questions from most adults such as "'How is school"? The child feels compelled to answer. Questions exaggerate the differential power between therapist and child. I have learned that a reflective observance of the child's play allows the child to decide what they wish the therapist to know. In this way, I became aligned to a child. I said to a 9-year-old, "you wanted to hide, maybe from me", which was so much more evocative than *where are you* or *why are you hiding?* Ginott (1968) wrote:

> *In play, a child can communicate ... hidden feelings, act out forbidden dramas, and rehearse and resolve interpersonal and intrapsychic dilemmas. The role of the therapist is to comprehend play language and to communicate his understanding to the child. The child's play messages, and the adult's verbal decoding become a healing dialogue. (p. 40)*

I was privileged to be a mentee of Ginott's student Arthur Orgel. Orgel trained a generation of psychiatry and psychology residents at the University of Rochester. Following in his mentor's footsteps, Orgel insisted that trainees clean up our playroom after our child patients, but he set this limit with a humorous non-offensive treatise which had a soft landing. True to Ginott, he worked to protect our experience with him as a trainer and supervisor.

Still, the question of the child's relationship with the therapist remained mysterious in my work. Winnicott's (1957) focus on attachment, and of bringing attachment into the work of a therapist with children brought an answer to the problem of the mothering therapist. Winnicott focused on attachment: of children to their parents, of child clients to their therapists, and the repair of attachments. He coined the term *good enough mother,* a more realistic view of parental possibilities, and the concept of holding, referring to the therapeutic space between patient and therapist. Winnicott posited that the creation of attachment occurs by the child experiencing mirroring, prizing, and *holding* (containing). These aspirations can become the basis for belonging in any relationship, and these foundations are less psychically laden than the earlier mothering therapist. Some examples of this from my practice, include the importance of greeting and making each child feel welcome, creating a sense of prizing, or, in the words of Mr. Rogers, communicating, *"You are special."*

Winnicott (1968) spoke of holding:

The consultant or specialist does not need to be clever so much as to be able to provide a natural and freely moving human relationship within the professional setting while the patient gradually surprises himself by the production of ideas and feelings that have not been previously integrated into the total personality. Perhaps the main work done is of the nature of integration, made possible by the reliance on the human but professional relationship---a form of 'holding. (p. 98)

I remember the natural and freely moving game a child patient came to love when we worked together. He had a complicated family, and a difficult stepfather. One of the objects for play in the office was a stuffed human form that he liked to throw around the room. One warm but pleasant day he discovered that he could open a window in my second-floor office. I debated whether to set a limit but wanted to see what he would do with the open window. Labeling the stuffed humanoid figure *stepfather,* he threw it out the window of my office repeatedly, session after session, running down the stairs to retrieve it and throwing it out once again. We both gained freedom from this play, as my wish to follow and witness his lead challenged me to become more flexible.

Winnicott also contributed the *squiggle game* to my play therapy repertoire, in which child and therapist both make a scribble, they then exchange scribbles and create something from it. The game is non-threatening, creates a kind of calming parallel, mirroring play between child and therapist, and allows the therapist to observe what the child projects: a snake? A bird? A dinosaur? An ice cream cone? Winnicott (1968) wrote:

It would go against my intention if the Squiggle game should become standardized or too clearly depicted. The principle is that psychotherapy is done in an overlap of the area of play of the child and the area of play of the adult or therapist. (p. 112)

The 70's and 80's created a different me with another lens for my work with children. During this time, Jacquelin Goldman introduced me to Piaget and Winnicott, who influenced my work. In Goldman's work, play therapy became the space in which the child could make the next developmental step, with the therapist helping the child overcome impediments to growth and providing the safety to do so. From the point of view of evolution of treatment approaches, Goldman moved play therapy out of the playroom, allowing the play to occur when the child and therapist were together. Goldman's approach also acknowledged the emotional impact *on the therapist* of the work with children. In other words, she addressed "the person of the therapist" (Goldman, 1968, p. 94). Goldman's influence on me and on my work evolved not just from her writing and powerful intellect, but also from the ways that we connected, over dinners, walks in nature, attending conferences. She modeled *growth in connection,* beyond the walls of her office.

My treatment of Shawna through play therapy is an example of my work as a therapist 15 years ago, standing on the shoulders of Ginott, Orgel, Winnicott, Goldman and others. Shawna had a history of medical trauma, traumatic loss, and sexual abuse. From my playroom sand tray, she selected a tiny wedding favor, a wedding cake filled with liquid bubbles. The bubbles became her most important element of play and eventually moved from the playroom to the lawn outside my office. Shawna loved creating bubbles, destroying them, and saving and protecting them. She grew past her trauma through experiencing in the context of her relationship with me. Through the bubble play she *experienced* joy. We *shared* joy.

I have continued to grow as a therapist since my work with Shawna. Training in family therapy added important tools. Raising and launching my own three children added humility and perspective, yet another depth to the work I have chosen and continue to choose. A still more recent case may illustrate my assimilation numerous techniques, and the resulting accommodation to a broader, more flexible form of therapy. It echoes Thoma and Cicero (2009) in its use of common factors, and, reflects both my intuition and my awareness of context.

Six-year-old Emma is the younger of two. She has a brother 3 years older, a successful professional mother who runs a family business and a father, a tradesman who also works in the family business. Emma's mother brought Emma into my office to address her sliding school performance, clinginess, and anxiety that were disrupting her sleep. Emma reluctantly released her mother in the waiting room and entered the playroom with me. I asked her to draw her family first, and she used only one brown marker to draw an anxious *floating* family. She then gravitated to the sand tray. She chose a pink Eiffel tower, a superhero, a lantern, strawberry shortcake, and a swing. Then with a huge sigh she added tiny beer cans and wine bottles and asked for her mother to join us. When her mother joined us, I asked Emma about the bottles, how they made her feel, and she replied that they "make dad yell and make kids feel sad and scared". She then climbed into her mother's lap, and together they rocked in the rocking chair, while the mother leaked quiet tears down her cheeks. I was sad with them, as I, too, have known the wounds from family addiction. which may have enabled me to be more present to their pain. Also, years of living and working have made me less critical or judgmental of parenting missteps—I have made many myself—and the absence of judgment always seems to make deeper emotions more accessible.

The next visit, after a few moments of exploring the playroom, I invited Emma to play the squiggle game. She drew lightning, a *spider horse,* a heart face, and a snake eating mouse; her themes of fear and anxiety were obvious in the drawings. Over the next session or two she let me in on some anxieties with her brother, with schoolwork, and her nightmares of spiders. We added some assertiveness skills through play for dealing with a "bossy" older brother. We talked and played through a technique for mastering nightmares. Emma painted and colored and talked through many anxieties and fears. And on a separate, child-free visit, her mother and I discussed Emma's dad's commitment to sobriety. The mother had been empowered through participation with Emma's sand tray to directly address the issue with her husband. No doubt, due to both changes in Emma and changes in the family, Emma's anxieties resolved. In our last visit, she drew another picture of her family, this time with everyone depicted in many colors. In Ginott style I said, "you wanted to show me how things are with your family". She said, "things are happier with dad, and my brother is nicer to me".

Play therapy has evolved, and I have evolved as a play therapist from the work I started with Eddie. I know the child within me well, by this point, and my years of work with children has been the most incredible training for seeing the child within so many of my adult clients. I have been richly blessed by teachers and supervisors, and by "paper teachers," writers and thinkers about play therapy, by my students, and by my young clients. I owe each of them a debt of gratitude, not only for development in my career, but also the personal development my career afforded me. As a therapist I have become stronger by trusting my own understanding and intuition. I know many theories but hold them loosely. I am more flexible and continue to be surprised by aspects of myself that show themselves in moments of play with a client. I delight in my work; a delight tempered with increasing bittersweetness.

I frequently walk across the bridge spanning the intracoastal waterway near my home. The nearest side of the bridge ascends steeply to the bridge's apex, then descends more gradually to the shore nearest the beach. When standing at the apex, looking toward home, the distance behind me is much longer than the steeper, shorter distance ahead. And so it is to be in one's 70s, when all that is behind is cumulatively greater than what is ahead. As I am nearing the end of my most active years in my career, I often wonder what might be next for the profession...

My former post-doctoral student, Dr. Kim Rust, gave me a glimpse of what might be next. She is fully loaded for technology, and passionate about her work with children and families. When COVID hit, she adapted with creativity. Her story follows, after these references.

References

Axline, V. (1947). *Play Therapy*. Ballantine Books.

Axline, V. (1964). *Dibs in search of self.* Ballantine Books.

Behan, D. (2022). Do clients train therapists to become eclectic and use the common factors? A qualitative study listening to experienced psychotherapists. *BMC Psychology,* 10(1), 183.

Ginott, Haim (1961). *Group psychotherapy with children: The theory and practice of play therapy.* McGraw-Hill.

Ginott, Haim (1968). Interpretations and child therapy. *Voices,* 4, 40-43.

Goldman, J. (1976). Becoming a psychotherapist. Charles Thomas.

Norton, P. (2009). A case of joy. *Voices,* 45. 3, 61-62.

Piaget, J. (1975). L'equilibration des structure cognitives. Probleme central du development. (Equilibration of cognitive structures. The central problem of cognitive development.) Presses de universitat de France.

Řiháček, T., & Danelova, E. (2016). The journey of an integrationist: A grounded theory analysis. *Psychotherapy,* 53(1), 78.

Řiháček, T., & Danelova, E. (2018). How Therapists Change: What motivates therapists towards integration? *European Journal for Qualitative Research in Psychotherapy,* 8, 1-12.

Rogers, C. (1951). *Client-centered therapy: Its current practice, implications, and theory.* Constable

Thoma, N. & Cecero, J. (2009). Is integrative use of techniques in psychotherapy the exception or the rule? Results of a national survey of doctoral level psychologists. *Psychotherapy,* 46(4), 405-417.

Winnicott, D.W. (1957). *The child and the family.* Tavistock.

Winnicott, D.W. (1968). The squiggle game. *Voices,* 4, 98-112.

Kim Rust

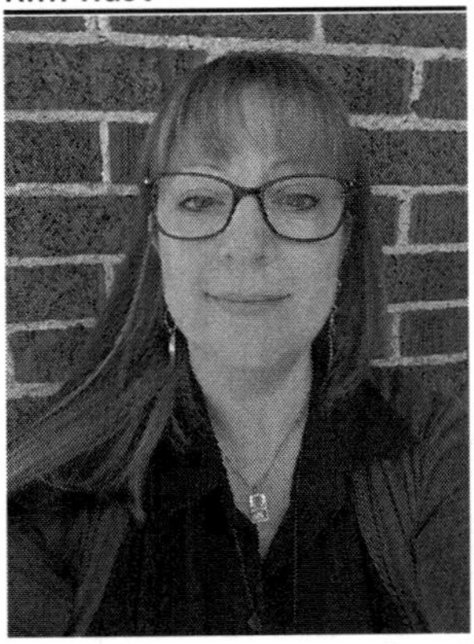

Kim Rust, PhD, practices clinical psychology in Deland, Florida. A 2021 graduate of Fielding Graduate University, she became licensed in Florida in 2022. Dr. Rust is also a Licensed Clinical Social Worker (LCSW) and has been in private practice since 2010. She has taught at Fielding University since May 2024. Dr. Rust approaches both counseling and assessment as healing processes, helping to answer deep-seated questions that individuals have about themselves or their child. She has a passion for providing LGBTQIA+ and Neurodiversity-affirming services. She was late-diagnosed as autistic, which may at least partially explain the abundant neurodiversity among her friends and family. When not working, she enjoys spending time with her husband, her two amazing children, and her kitten, Freyja. She loves reading supernatural books, since the problems in those stories are nothing like the real world. *kimrustphd@gmail.com*

Necessity is the Mother of Invention:
Virtual Play Therapy Office

In the Fall of 2022, I had the great privilege and joy to engage in post-doctoral work under the mentorship of Dr. Penelope Norton and to spend my days with children in her beautiful play therapy room. The warmth of her playroom and her amazing collection of toys cannot be overstated. Imagine a giant sand tray, huge dollhouse, walls of carefully selected figurines, a myriad of puppets, and an extensive collection of authentic Troll dolls. Classic toys from every decade for the last 40+ years invite a rich and engaging experience for children.

By harsh contrast, in July of 2020, just months into the COVID-19 pandemic, I moved my family to Missouri for my doctoral internship year, only to spend the first eight months conducting therapy sessions via Zoom (aka TeleHealth). TeleHealth was not my favorite. I once quipped that, when doing TeleHealth, I felt like a "cat without its whiskers," since I was missing so much salient information: the emotional temperature in the room, the natural flow of conversation (which were often complicated by technology glitches), or even clues about my client's hygiene that day. No doubt my clients were missing significant information about me as well—like subtle changes in posture to show my interest or subtle shifts in the crinkles around my eyes to show shared sadness or humor, blurred out by Zoom filters.

TeleHealth worked pretty well for my teen and adult clients, but was much, much more difficult for my child clients. I still remember a disastrous session early on with one little boy*, who was struggling in the aftermath of his parents' divorce and being stuck at home during a global pandemic. Whereas in person, I could follow him around the playroom and talk to him while engaging in more physical activities, my efforts to speak to him at length fell flat. He stopped responding to my questions and began simply rolling around (and off of!) the bed where the iPad had been placed. He knocked a lamp on the floor. My efforts to call him back to our conversation were futile, and I felt I was wasting everyone's time.

I had been trained as a play therapist, both in nondirective play and in The Play Project (a DIR-Floortime-inspired intervention that helps adults cultivate joyful engagement with autistic children). Sitting in separate rooms and across miles, I missed the easy engagement with young children with the toys and art supplies in my playroom. In play therapy, following the child's lead is essential. When I tried to do this over basic TeleHealth, my efforts often disintegrated into the child restlessly roaming around the room. I could have the child draw a picture (using materials they had at home), for example, but I was unable to visually see the process of their drawing and therefore could not effectively reflect and mirror that back to them. And when I tried to talk to the young children about how they were doing, I often hit a developmental wall and lost their interest. Even if they were precocious and able to articulate their experiences, it did not serve to treat them as "mini adults"—children need to express their emotions and work through their experiences more holistically, using movement, play, and art. Perhaps as much to make my life easier as to help the children I served, I decided to create a virtual play therapy room.

Looking back, I wish I could give credit to the original virtual office that I modified, but the source of that excellent template is lost deep in the bizarre time lapse that was 2020. Currently, you can find YouTube videos that walk you through process (e.g., Google "How to Create a Bitmoji Therapy Room"), and I am happy to share my template with anyone that wants it. The basis is Google Slides, which is something like PowerPoint. You represent online links with images in your office (e.g., the sandbox represents the virtual sand tray activity). You have the ability to include a personalized cartoon of yourself (the Bitmoji). In "Presentation Mode," you can share these slides with your client. In my experience, it works best in Zoom because you can share mouse control and sound, so the child client can click using their mouse or tablet to select the next activity. This brings back the child-led element that is missing from typical TeleHealth with children.

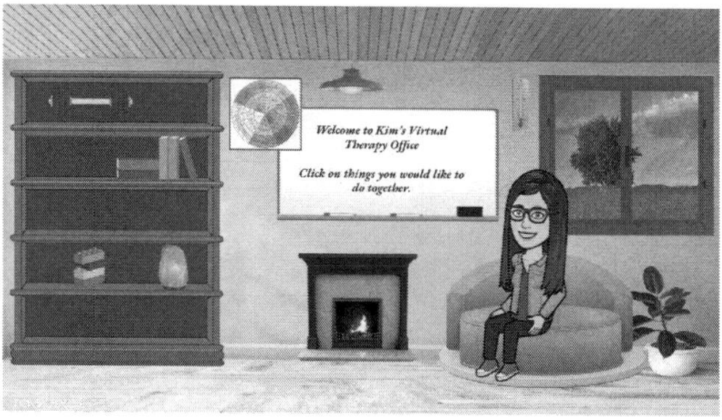

My virtual play therapy office has a "waiting room," which includes a link to views from windows all over the world and four other rooms: a playroom, a relaxation room, a reading room, and an exercise room. The reading room has links for YouTube videos reading various children's books aloud. The exercise room has dance and exercise videos. More complex activities are found in the playroom and relaxation room. For example, the playroom includes a virtual dollhouse and sandtray, as well as art and

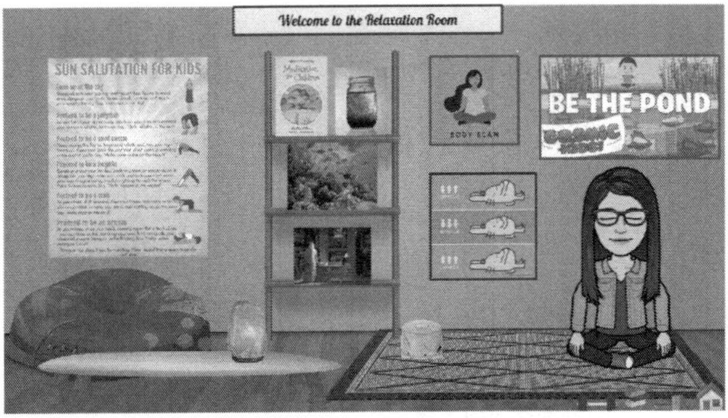
Welcome to the Relaxation Room
SUN SALUTATION FOR KIDS
BODY SCAN
BE THE POND

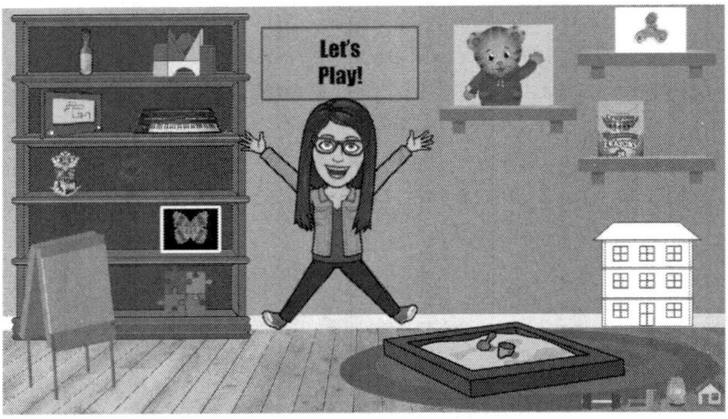
Let's Play!

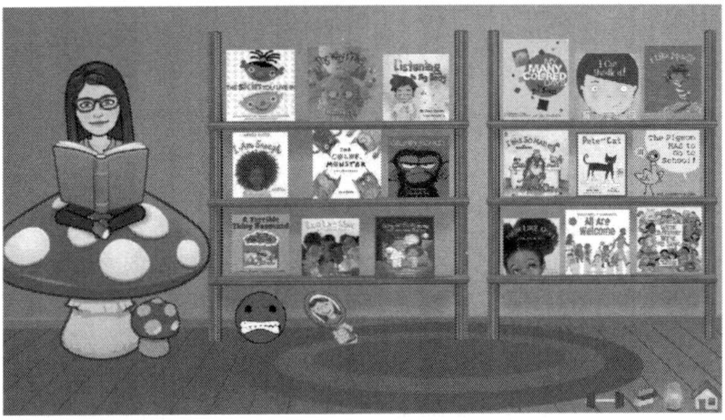
Pete the Cat
The Pigeon HAS to Go to School!
All Are Welcome

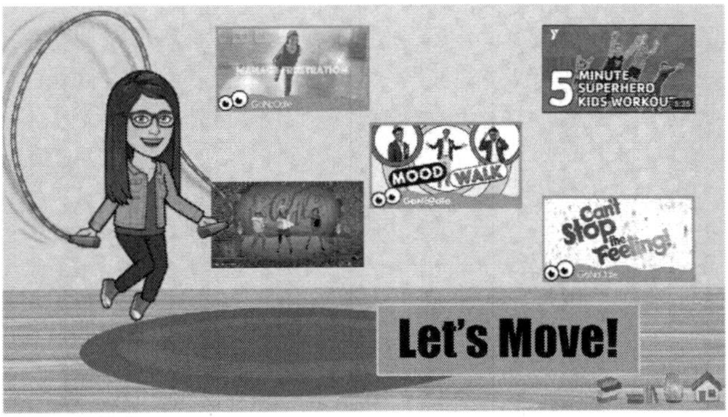
5 MINUTE SUPERHERO KIDS WORKOU
MOOD WALK
Can't Stop the Feeling!
Let's Move!

music activities. The relaxation room may be my genuine favorite. It includes several guided meditations, a close-up video of glitter settling in a glitter jar, an underwater video of fish swimming, and a video of Dumbledore's office with soothing music from the world of Harry Potter.

"...I would encourage any clinician who works with children to spend a few hours creating a virtual play therapy office."

One child's use of the virtual dollhouse was particularly poignant. Ellie,* a 7-year-old with a delicate frame and an ethereal air, still grieved the mother she could not recall, who had died suddenly when she was two years old. Though raised by a devoted father, with substantial extended family support, Ellie often asked her father when he was "going to get her a new Mommy" and expressed sadness and envy when she witnessed even mundane family activities, such as families with two parents eating dinner at a restaurant. In the virtual dollhouse, Ellie was able to show me her "dream house," which included both her father and mother, as well as her and a dog. She had the family members interact lovingly, with the mother figure being particularly sweet and loving to the daughter figure. Then she showed me her "real house," with just her and her father. She showed herself and her father also interacting lovingly, spending time together playing board games and talking about her life and feelings. Through this virtual play, I was able to help Ellie to reflect on the many positives of her "real house," even if her "dream house" was not something within her reach.

Angie* was a particularly anxious child whom I saw during this time, who followed my suggestion to try out activities in the relaxation room. Angie had many siblings, all piled in the house together during lockdown, but she would retreat to a tiny linen closet for our sessions. We would sit together and engage in guided meditations telling us to "be the pond" while the fish rippled the water around us. We would listen to peaceful music while watching a camera pan around Dumbledore's office. I remember Angie sighing at one point, with her eyes fixed on the peaceful images on the screen, and saying, "It is just so quiet here." I could feel my own breathing slow, and myself tune into how the anxiety seemed to flow away from both of us. In the height of the stress of the COVID-19 pandemic, sitting with a child while we watched glitter settle or the fish swim felt truly healing.

One might question the benefits of such a virtual office. To be honest, I would not choose the virtual office over in-person play therapy. It cannot bring in the depth of the unspoken connection between therapist and client that in-person work allows. The activities are also limited and do not have the tactile element in a "real" playroom. However, I do consider it a viable alternative when in-person sessions are not possible (e.g., during the pandemic, or currently, if a child or caregiver is sick or otherwise unable to make the appointment in-person).

Technology is a medium that children are quite comfortable with, and as long as the family has a computer or touchscreen tablet and an internet connection, this option is fairly accessible.

Some considerations also apply to general TeleHealth in terms of safety. If a child has a tendency to become quite dysregulated or has serious trauma, the clinician may want to be more directive to help monitor and contain how the child was feeling during the virtual session. In addition, collaboration with parents or caregivers to ensure that they process afterwards with the child could be quite important.

In general, I would encourage any clinician who works with children to spend a few hours creating a virtual play therapy office. It is a fun and useful tool to have in one's back pocket should the need arise.

**The cases described have been modified to protect the children's identities. Necessity is the Mother of Invention: Virtual Play Therapy Office*

Commentary

"Plus ca change, plus c'est la meme chose."

Indeed, the more things change, the more they stay the same. These two articles reflect the evolution of both child therapy and the person of the child therapist. As I read them both, I reflected on my own development as a therapist and a person over a 45 year career, and I must admit that I was fortunate to have ceased practice immediately prior to Covid and the profound disruption that that ushered in. The prospect of doing child therapy over Zoom still seems daunting to me and I commend the author/therapist who made a creative solution to this dilemma. I'm sure she was not taught this in graduate school, but rather developed this out of necessity. Bravo! I do note some commonalities salient to both articles. These perhaps are the core of all good therapy regardless of theoretical orientation or approach.

In my view, the starting point is the connection between the therapist and the patient—relationship is primary. Clearly both of these authors value this characteristic above any theory or pragmatic approach. In this context, empathic understanding whether explicitly spoken or enacted is key for the connection. Equally important is authenticity. In my experience, kids have a remarkable ability to perceive 'fakiness' and know when they are truly 'seen'. It is critically important to acknowledge and accept the experience of the child as much as possible without judgment. Since underlying much distress, whether trauma, developmental problems, or constitutional/temperamental traits, is most succinctly described as aloneness in one's suffering; connecting and accepting the totality of the other is paramount. Both authors seem to grasp this with clarity and certainty. Woven through this fabric is the need for tolerance of ambiguity and 'not knowing' as much of play therapy is nonlinear and even, at times, free form and mysterious. In short, the therapist must be flexible and open to the sometimes surreal.

Both authors have had the good fortune to have had excellent training and the luxury of supportive, engaging mentors. This reflects my tenet that the relationship is the starting point and core of healing and growth. It is true for therapy and it is equally true for supervision- the child patient and the child therapist both grow when nurtured. These two articles serve as a reminder that the field is constantly evolving and requires creativity to adapt to changing ideas and circumstances. Although I am now some years past practicing, I found both articles engaging and thought provoking. I am left with wanting to know more about each author's internal experience of these changes and their reflections on their own evolution and adaptations, and that seems like a good take away—more curiosity and a desire for more personal connection.

—Z Rosenzweig, PhD

"It is a huge danger to pretend that awful things do not happen.
But you need enough hope to keep on going.
I am trying to make hope."
— Corita Kent 1918-1986

Commentary

I admired and learned a lot from what Penelope Norton, PhD, and Kim Rust, PhD shared with us. I also appreciate the view of generativity in action, as Penelope Norton describes the evolution of play therapy that seems embedded in the kind of virtual play therapy room that Kim Rust described creating and holding for her child clients through the Covid-19 pandemic. It gives me hope that the wisdom of the past will live on and not be lost to the technological change of the present, and that assimilation and accommodation will continue.

Penelope Norton, demonstrated the courage and humility to grow and keep on growing over the course of her years as a child therapist. I like the idea that patients might teach us to discern the common factors of psychotherapy, but to move from model to model to beyond models is not easy, and requires us to work in a state of uncertainty for extended periods. I really appreciated the walk through the development of play therapy, and the way Kim Rust internalized it and incorporated it into her virtual play therapy space. I admired Penelope Norton's commitment to wrestling with the various theories that came out during or soon before her training. In my own training, much of psychodynamic or humanistic-oriented play therapy had been supplanted by cognitive-behavioral play therapy. In this model, play is a medium for teaching particular skills, like in the relaxation room that Kim Rust describes. The model also is more therapist-led than client-led, which didn't sit well with me. Cognitive behavioral play therapy loses some (but not all) of the symbolic communication in the play, but still can lead to the kinds of mastery over strong emotions and traumatic experiences that Norton and Rust describe.

For me, the cognitive behavioral model always felt a little too prescriptive, impersonal, and superficial. I used to joke about the method in a frame that comes from my Catholic upbringing: "Take 5 deep breaths and 3 progressive muscle relaxations, and go forth and be anxious no more." But it did highlight for me the importance of what happens in the therapy room needs to extend beyond the therapy room, and that the therapeutic relationship is necessary but not always a sufficient means of change for the client.

I also admire the challenge that Penelope Norton described in sitting with a senior male supervisor focusing on oedipal issues of a client towards her uncle when her inner understanding of the patient was to believe the patient who said that her uncle had sexually assaulted her. I would have liked to hear more about how she resolved that silent internal wrestling with herself and with her supervisor, as it sounds to me like the seeds of developing her own powerful voice as a therapist.

I particularly liked her analysis of how her own parenting and the struggles and countertransference that arise from taking different stances changed the way she engaged with children over time. I remember in my own practice some very helpful moments of supporting unrestricted play in my clients and one particularly disastrous one. I was working with a 10-year-old boy and we went out to explore the woods next to my office. We came to a ditch that went down about 4 feet which started about 2 feet wide but widened as it went further along. My client started jumping over the ditch and then going to wider places. He made the first two jumps, before I gently cautioned him that the third jump he was going to try seemed pretty far. He went for it anyway, fell in the ditch, twisted his ankle, and cried out in a lot of pain. I ended up taking him out on my back, so we both got back to my office muddied, disheveled, and him still crying in a lot of pain. His parents took him to the ER and let me know that he had a sprain and was going to be fine, but that was the last time I saw this client. I certainly wished that I had been better at setting limits to keep him safe, and I think he and his parents wished the same thing.

In reading Kim Rust's article, I felt a little awed by the care, thought, creativity, and commitment that I imagine it took to create the virtual play therapy space online for her child clients. One of the things so many therapists spoke of during the pandemic was how challenging it was to work with people while both they and their clients were going through this shared trauma of a deadly virus. It seems that Dr. Rust did not allow her own emotional reactions to the pandemic hold her back from trying to be as present as possible in helping her child patients. During the pandemic, I saw some younger clients whom I simply could not keep on the screen for sessions: I just gave up, moving the work to parent-child or family therapy so that the parent(s) could help keep the child on task and engaged, and I raised the age of clients I saw. I wish I had the creativity, savviness with technology, and gumption to follow in Kim Rust's footsteps: my child clients would have been better off for it.

I really appreciated Kim Rust's description of being "a cat without whiskers" in working online with individuals, especially children. I too have experienced some loss of a sense of connection, sometimes from something as basic as being unable to really look someone in the eye. However, I think it's important to recognize some of the distinctive strengths of online therapy as well. First of all, while I see less of people's whole bodies, I can see more of the micro-expressions on people's faces in virtual therapy. Second, I think we can gain more insight into our clients' real-world conditions when they are in their homes during sessions. Sometimes, for instance, I can hear the arguing or chaos that a kid is responding to in the home environment that I would have no way of experiencing directly in the in-person work, since we would be in my office and not in the home.

—Matthew Leary PhD

THIS

Katherine Williams

kjwilliamsphd@gmail.com

It's this particular moment
when the cave of sleep still
calls and stale years linger
in stifling air when
the slick black window
glares it's habit that opens
the door to the waiting day
and this particular slip
of light through the frothy cedar
that hides a mourning dove
whose dusky ancestors crooned
as moons paled and whose children's
children may cooa coo coo coo
through shining branches
as long as this world survives.

Last Swallow

Katherine Williams

in memory of my mother, paralyzed as a young woman

It was never too early to creep
To the white sheeted room where she lay.
As if from inside her private waking
She'd make a space just wide enough
To let me in to watch first light
Glide along the sill. The last swallow
Of water in her bedside glass, silver
For a minute. Juniper's green breath
Against the window. Milk in clear bottles
Delivered to the other side of the wall.

If asked, I'd have said we had conversations.
But what I remember of those mornings
Is the lush new day ahead of us,
The hush of her long still body, listening.

Sorrows

Katherine Williams

after Lucille Clifton

who would believe them old
yet still fierce

their bony fingers nearly stopping breath
in the middle of a petaled day

lifting off layers of time until
only the bruised center

remains   who would believe
they know to set language adrift

above deserts and city streets
consonants clicking softly

vowels going out like waves
while all the while the stiff fingers

tenderly gather us in
from rooms, from rubble

to touch and breathe
together

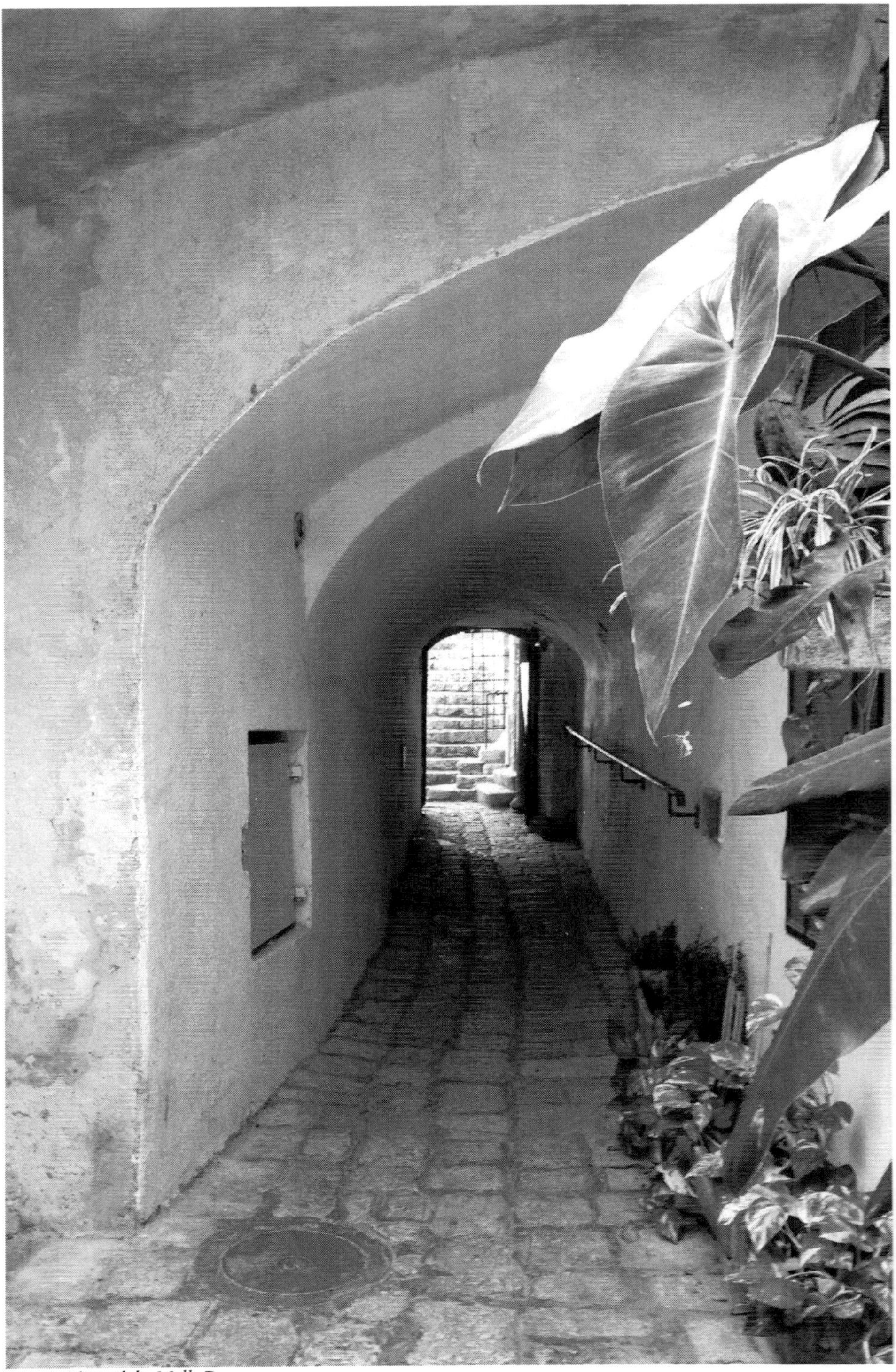

Passing Through by Molly Donovan

Jerry Gans

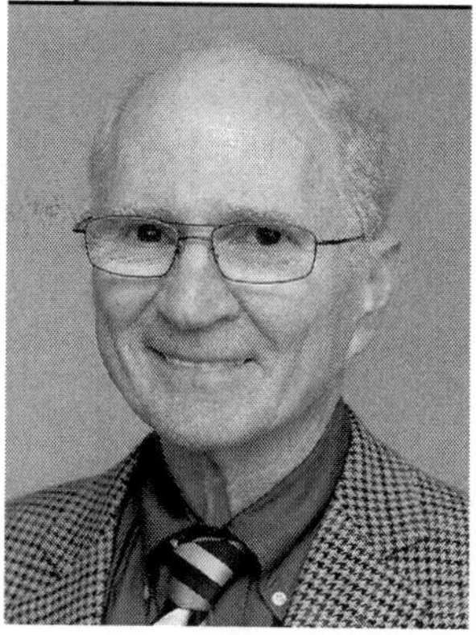

Jerry Gans, MD has been married for 61 years and has three daughters and five grandchildren. He is a Distinguished Life Fellow of both the American Group Psychotherapy Association and American Psychiatric Association. An Associate Clinical Professor of Psychiatry, Harvard Medical School, Jerry retired in 2019 after 48 years of practice. The author of two books and over 50 refereed articles, book chapters and book reviews newspaper articles, Jerry has published widely on group and individual psychotherapy, psychological aspects of physical rehabilitation, liaison psychiatry, and psychotherapy and literature. In 2018, the Northeastern Society for Group Psychotherapy recognized his contributions with a Lifetime Achievement Award.

Dr. Elvin Semrad: A Memorable Teacher

THOUSANDS OF YEARS AGO, OR SO IT SEEMED, IN that far off kingdom of Cambridge, Massachusetts, 28 aspiring psychiatrists, I among them, trudged to that grubby font of learning known as the Mass Mental Health Center (MMHC) in Boston to begin our three-year psychiatric residency. The year was 1968. We came to learn from many distinguished psychiatrists, pre-eminent among them being Dr. Elvin Semrad. His corpulent, mustached, silver-haired Buddha-like presence had already presided over the education of a generation of psychiatrists, many of them no longer with us. He had an amazing ability to reduce complex life challenges to simple ideas expressed in ordinary language. In the first year of residency, we were exposed to his teachings at weekly case conferences where the residents took turns presenting their hospitalized patients, many of them recovering from psychotic episodes. First, the patient's history would be presented by the psychiatric resident, the social worker on the case, by the psychologist if there had been psychological testing, the nursing staff and any volunteers who had known the patient. Semrad would then interview the patient and after the interview, with the patient in the room if he/she chose to be, Dr. Semrad would talk about how we might be of help to patient. He took these occasions to offer pithy statements on a variety of topics: the body; the centrality of feelings; love; growing; maturing and sadness; leaving home; work; belief; thinking; decision making; happiness; and general remarks on life: Here are few of my favorites (Rako & Mazer, 1980.)

- What is there in life if you can't feel it in your body...love, joy, sadness, despair?
- The one thing all people have is feelings—their actions and thoughts are often a means of disguising these feelings from themselves.
- Falling in love is the only acceptable psychosis.
- One of the saddest things in life to accept is that those you love often love others more.
- The more mature a relationship, the more able the two people are to give up their dependency and learn how to live alone together.
- It's disillusioning to be mamma's fair-haired boy and then find out that the rest of the world doesn't treat you that way. It can scare the life out of you.
- You've got to love your patients.
- When you feel nothing, that's when you hurt the most.

Here are some of my memories of Dr. Semrad from my three years at the MMHC:

His pervasive presence –

During one September night of my first year of residency, I was Doctor on Call for the hospital. I was called up to Service I to see a 28-year-old woman who had been a patient of the Chief Resident for two years. Over that time, she had been hospitalized several times and knew the workings of the hospital inside and out. I was asked to evaluate the patient's request for sleeping medication. In those days, before the supremacy of biological psychiatry, we were taught that we were the medicine and the patient was the text, a text that we should know from cover to cover. Still new to the system, my evaluation of the request for medication could easily have been mistaken for a complete patient work-up.

Still very new to psychiatry, and feeling quite insecure, I did what many of the new residents did. We imitated Semrad, hoping that by using some of his simple language, we too could be effective with our patients.

The patient's room was dark and in a far corner she was curled up on her bed in fetal position. After about 25 minutes of asking her every question that I could pull out of my still small bag of tricks and getting absolutely nowhere, I decided that it was time to pull out all the stops and ask her a Semrad-like question. So I asked her, "Tell me, what is breaking your heart?" From across the dark room came the sharp retort, "Don't give me any of that Semrad shit!"

I immediately got up from my chair, went to the nurses' station and told them, "Give her whatever she wants for sleep."

Exposure to him at teaching conferences and what and how he taught us

At the first case conference chaired by Dr. Semrad that I had ever attended, a fellow resident was presenting the case of Mr. Jones, a man with an involutional depression [a diagnosis no longer used, referring to a depression resulting from developmental or hormonal changes of middle age and beyond—Editors] who was also alcoholic. In the discussion of the case after Dr. Semrad had interviewed the patient, and wanting to make a good first impression on Dr. Semrad, I offered the comment that the wives of alcoholics sometimes aid and abet their husband's drinking. I remember being brought up short by Dr. Semrad's reply, "If Mr. Jones's wife behaved that way, she is the first woman that I am aware of to do so." I worried that I had not gotten off to an auspicious start with Dr. Semrad.

In December of my first year of residency, I presented a 14-year-old-patient of mine to Dr. Semrad at a teaching conference. The young man was torn apart by the separation and divorce of his parents that occurred when he was five. His father ran off with the babysitter leaving the patient's borderline mother with four young children to care for and to raise. Shunted back and forth between his parents, the patient distracted and comforted himself by drawing cartoons. At the teaching conference, while I was telling Dr. Semrad about the young man, his cartoons were passed around to the clinicians in attendance. They became so engrossed in the cartoons that it became apparent in the discussion after Dr. Semrad's interview with the patient that many of the residents had not listened to the facts of the presentation. I remember Semrad cautioning the residents not to become more interested in a patient's productions than in the patient him or herself.

"Dr. Semrad also taught us not to gratify ourselves at the patient's expense. In my case, I think Dr. Semrad noticed that I was more invested in getting his approval than I was in the patient's welfare."

Dr. Semrad also taught us not to gratify ourselves at the patient's expense. In my case, I think Dr. Semrad noticed that I was more invested in getting his approval than I was in the patient's welfare. This realization was brought home to me when I presented to him at a teaching conference a 32-year-old, married woman who had tried to kill herself by overdosing. She showed little interest in learning about herself in therapy and even less interest in attending a teaching conference where she would be interviewed by the attending psychiatrist who, in her case, happened to be Dr. Semrad. The interview was noteworthy for how little we learned about the patient because she was quite guarded and only superficially cooperative. After the interview, Dr. Semrad turned to me and asked me how I had to prostitute myself to get the patient to come in for the interview. I learned a lot from that question.

Many of the questions that Dr. Semrad asked patients at case conferences, often the first question he asked them, had to do with how people do business with each other. It was the language of the market place, something I could easily relate to because my father had been a middleman in the fruit business. To the hospitalized manic patient whose behavior left his therapist no alternative but to hospitalize him, the question might be, "Did you get what you came for?" To the patient who had been alienated from her family for many years, the question might be, "How did you afford that?"

His answers to questions that patients asked him were illuminating as well. One answer I remember distinctly was in response to a question asked him by a 21-year-old man, "When is it time for a person to leave home?" Semrad's answer: "When the person is ready to."

"Semrad was deceptively relentless in his curiosity about the circumstances in which people made these decisions, decisions that in some instances would last a lifetime.

In his interviews with patients, Dr. Semrad demonstrated that we should not be overly puzzled by the trivial event that apparently precipitated a patient's psychotic break. Instead, he encouraged us to understand as fully as possible the patient's pre-morbid functioning and his/her character structure before the break occurred. Perhaps it only took a trivial occurrence to cause the decompensation because, in fact, the patient was barely holding things together before the precipitating event.

Dr. Semrad also exposed in his interviews the myth that some patients are empty. His interviews showed how the apparent emptiness was a defense, an avoidance of the profound feelings that were part of the internal conflict with which patients were struggling.

About feelings

The kinds of questions that Dr. Semrad asked patients gave me the impression that Dr. Semrad believed that people did not simply feel feelings but decided which feelings they would feel or if they would let themselves feel anything at all. "When did you decide to turn off your feelings?" was a question that Dr. Semrad asked a patient he was interviewing during a case conference, a patient who could only provide thoughts but no feelings.

Semrad was deceptively relentless in his curiosity about the circumstances in which people made these decisions, decisions that in some instances would last a lifetime. A few of my teachers at MMHC at the time were skeptical of this approach that they felt Dr. Semrad carried to an extreme. I remember one of these teachers wondering if Dr. Semrad would ask a patient, "When did you decide to develop rheumatoid arthritis?"

About making basic decisions in life

Dr. Semrad, in addition to being empathic and incredibly in touch with feelings of sadness, loneliness, and disappointment, was tough and tenacious. He was relentless in holding patients and staff alike responsible for making the decisions we all need to make in our lives. Treating patients and staff alike in this regard reflected his deep belief that people are much more similar than different. He felt, with regard to life's important tasks, that psychotic people and neurotic people were different only quantitatively, not qualitatively. He kept his eye on the ball; it was difficult, ultimately, to evade his questions. He was keenly aware of the difference between idealization and realistically valuing someone: as he once put it, "Don't idealize anyone, they all stink. But do realistically value people for what they have to offer."

I imagine that if he were alive today he would caution others not to idealize him. I can think of two groups that probably wouldn't. Psychopharmacologists would point out that Semrad's skepticism—or was it cynicism—about the efficacy of psychotropic drugs was rather extreme. Feminists would find his experience of women as limited, antiquated, possibly even condescending. Perhaps it was his Nebraska upbringing in the early 20th century and his Catholic faith that he practiced his entire life that contributed to his view of women as mainly loving, nurturing, non-competitive, and, above all, domestic.

Three of the most important things I learned from Dr. Semrad

Three of the most important things I learned about psychotherapy during my psychiatric residency, I learned from Dr. Semrad.

The first was respect for the patient. During every case conference that Dr. Semrad chaired, and immediately after he was done interviewing the patient, he would ask the patient, "Do I have your permission to talk with these doctors, nurses and social workers about how we might best be of help to you?" I recall how profoundly this question affected me. Here we were, a group of highly successful professionals and there was the patient, often a broken-down person saturated with feelings of failure and shame, and here was Dr. Semrad extending to the patient such respect.

The second thing I learned was to always wonder what it might be about me that was keeping certain dimensions of the patient from surfacing, from finding expression in the therapy hour or during the hospital stay. How did Dr. Semrad teach us that? Repeatedly, we residents would watch him interview a patient at a clinical conference – a patient that we had been working with for several months—only to find the patient telling Semrad things that the patient had never told us. Once or twice, the patients' revelations might be a matter of chance. But seeing this phenomenon happen over and over again made it virtually impossible for us not to wonder, "What is it about us that keeps our patients from telling us this highly personal information?" What are we unwittingly doing to impede the very enterprise we are trying to advance?"

And last but not least was to value my own personal experience. When we came to MMHC fresh out of internship, we were probably as smart as we would ever be. We had just finished a year of medical or pediatric internship, using our vast knowledge to take care of patients, only to walk on to a psychiatric in-patient unit where most of our knowledge would be of little use in helping severely ill mental patients. It was very upsetting and frightening for us. It was at that juncture that Semrad said something that I have always treasured: "The one thing that each of you has that no one else has is your own experience as you experienced it. You might not like it, you may feel it stinks, you may not have elected it; but it is yours, SO VALUE AND USE IT." At a time when our knowledge of the theory and practice of psychotherapy was minimal, it was so reassuring to have a person in authority tell us that our personal experience was valuable and that we should us it.

I vividly remember being part of an instantly bereaved community when news of Dr. Semrad's sudden death at the age of 66 on July 1, 1976 reverberated through his "psychotherapy offspring." It was as if, in the moment, we had all lost a beloved mother and father combined in one person.

Reference

Rako, S. & Mazer, H. (1980). *Semrad: The Heart of a Therapist.* New York and London: Jason Aronson.

Commentary:

The author gives us a wonderfully vivid portrayal of both his mentor, and his own experiences as a novice psychiatric trainee, and I am sure I would have benefitted from getting to know either of them. The way the piece is written enables us to see both the positive and negative potential in Dr. Semrad's framing of psychological defenses as a choice. On the one hand, it may be empowering and liberating, showing patients that they have more responsibility and freedom than they realized for their internal dynamics. On the other hand, it can be distancing and judgmental to contradict patients' lived experiences; it can lead to either more self-blame in the already depressed, or to frank hostility to the therapist who dishes out "that Semrad-shit."

There were also definitely places in the article where I found myself marveling at the young trainee's determination to extract wisdom and clinical skill from what came across to me as slapdash and even self-indulgent behavior from Semrad. For instance, it sounded to me like he wanted to blame the young author for presenting a patient who frustrated Semrad, or made him look like a poor interviewer. The author -- wide eyed and trusting -- turned it into a learning experience for himself, by taking a fresh look at his interactions with the patient, but as a reader, I'm not as ready to credit Semrad's teaching here.

Lastly, I find the author so deft in the gentle way he addresses his doubts about Semrad's limitations concerning medication and female psychology—direct, but balanced and nonjudgmental—that I find myself instinctively trusting him as a psychotherapist. The fact that he has retired is a loss to our professional community, but I am grateful that he still writes for us.

—Jonathan Farber

Barry J. Wepman

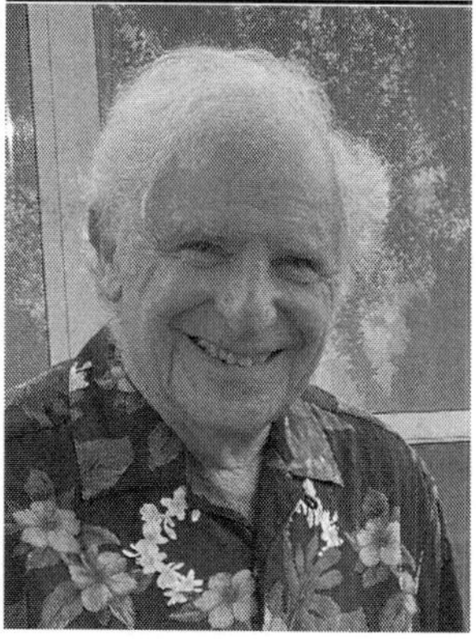

Barry Wepman has been an academy member since 1980. In his early years he chaired the Eastern regional group, was on EC, and ran many groups, workshops, and training institutes, and also chaired the program for several national meetings. He is delighted to see that such institutionally important jobs are being picked up with enthusiasm by more recent members. It gives him hope for the future to be in the backdraft of the energy of the newer generations.

A Song of Appreciation

In 1976, I was a newly minted PhD psychologist working in the psychiatry department of a medical school and trying to figure out how to have a practice in psychotherapy. I'd wound up there by accident. The post-doc I'd arranged at Boston State Hospital had been defunded when I'd had just months to go before I was to get my degree, and I found (desperate) respite in an academic job in New York, where I was also able to do a year of training in family and couples therapy. After a year, a much better (and more secure) job came up across the river at the University of Medicine and Dentistry of New Jersey, so I grabbed it. While I was glad to be there, the faculty members around me were a typical mix of community psychiatry types: behaviorists, psychopharmacologists, and one Rogerian. None of these folks operated from a map that made sense in the ways I thought about the terrain of therapy. I felt in search of a role model and of a theory base and a style of practice that fit me. I joke that I had dropped out of psychology several times, since I'd tried—in high school, college, and even a first attempt at graduate school—to learn a form of psychology that made sense to me. What I'd found were people doing something far different from what I'd conceptualized, and they had a certainty about their methods that put me off.

I'd been in therapy for a while in Boston, before all this, with a therapist who'd felt very effective to me. He'd left a job in the VA system having lost faith in psychotherapy, had done research for a while, and then spent some time at Esalen, where he'd discovered how psychotherapy could work. I would say he used some

"...my longest standing mentor relationship in the Academy is with my family group. I can't say enough about the way the members have held me, confronted me, and influenced the way I've practiced psychotherapy.

combination of psychodynamic and Gestalt techniques. In today's parlance his method would probably be called relational, but that had been many years before that designation existed in the world of therapy. Looking back, I think that that's what I'd been searching for.

Now I was with people who were a bit closer to this conceptualization, but still off the mark. I knew what didn't feel good, although what didn't feel good to me seemed to have had a lot of currency in the worlds I'd found. So, likely, it was that prior therapist's approach that I was looking for.

On the other hand, maybe it was about my mother. My mother was a caring and sensitive person. Several of the neighborhood kids used to come and talk to her when they had things to discuss, and I guess you could call her manner relational, too. At any rate I didn't see anything like that in the medical school.

My department ran a program designed for the psychiatry residents in which a practitioner from the community would present a video-recorded session and then discuss what he/she had been doing or thinking during the session. I kept attending these presentations, but didn't see anything that worked for me until at last, deep into the spring, I saw one that hit. The presenter's style was rather unorthodox, as a therapist he seemed human, spontaneous, and a bit off the wall. I was impressed, not only by his work, but also by his willingness to display it in front of an audience of academics who were quite different from him. The next week I called Harry Rockberger and asked him to lunch.

Harry and I had many lunches and meetings in his office over the next months while I jumped through the hoops necessary to qualify for professional licensure. Our conversations were about the realities of psychotherapy practice, about theory (or lack thereof), about self-care. When I got my license, I asked Harry if I could use his office a few hours a week as I started my practice. He said I could, on the condition that I join The American Academy of Psychotherapists. Anxious to be able to use his office I agreed, although, in truth, I had no idea what I was getting into. It turns out that Harry had been a graduate school friend of Henry Guze and Jules Barron, two of the founders of the Academy, and had been an AAP member since a year or two after its inception.

My first AAP event was a weekend conference of the Northeast Regional Affiliate. It took place on Long Island, and I don't remember much about it other than that I met Jerry Travers and Mark Stern, two long-time members, and that they seemed to take a shine to me. It was all pretty confusing. Jerry lived one town over from me in New Jersey, and over the next months we met frequently. He helped me in more ways than I can recount. It was he that convinced me to go to my first national event, the 1981 I&C in New York City. At that meeting Jerry took me in hand and began to introduce me to people who over the years have had a great influence both on my person and on the way, I think of and practice psychotherapy. Mark, who had been Jerry's therapist, was editor of *Voices,* and within a year of my entry into the Academy invited me onto the editorial board—quite an honor at that time.

I was disoriented by the regard in which these esteemed men seemed to hold me.

My father had had a childhood of poverty, terror, and abandonment. His father had come to the US, leaving his family to wait in Latvia until he'd been able to send passage money. In the meantime, his mother and younger sister had died, leaving a family of four children with no parents to make their way across the ocean to the US. He was an anxious and critical person, and I was not accustomed to the positive regard of older men, so I was warmed, but wary, of what I was getting. The idea of mentorship seemed unattainable.

One of the first pieces I was asked to review for *Voices* was an article written by Dugald Arbuckle, the then president of AAP. He, too, was a large figure in the Academy and in the field, having been the chairman of the psychology department at Boston University. In those days *Voices* didn't use blind review procedures; the identities of writer and reviewer were known to each other, and the writer was given a (signed) copy of the reviewer's evaluation. I remember reading the article, first with excitement, and, then, with growing alarm. I found what I felt were flaws in reasoning, logical inconsistencies, and grammatical errors. "What to do?" I thought. It was my first assignment, it was from the president of this new (to me) organization of experienced therapists, and I was thinking of recommending against publishing it. I called Jerry and presented my dilemma and he said a version of, "Mark put you on the editorial board because he trusted your judgment." I bit the bullet, and, with trepidation, submitted a kind, but detailed, review with the recommendation to "reject as submitted."

A short time later I received a new copy of Dugald's piece, which incorporated most of the suggestions I'd made, accompanied by a note from the author thanking me for my comments, and telling me that he felt the article was much improved for my efforts. I was relieved, felt appreciated, and thought, "these are people I can live with."

Fast forward to another time in my life, a time of great personal pain and struggle. I sought out Sol Rosenberg. Sol, another one-time president of the Academy, was a revered person in our organization. I'd known him for five years, or so, loved him, and felt respected by him in a way that, again, contradicted the voice I'd internalized from my father. Sol was a wise, kind, open, brave man. I had first become aware of him when, in 1981, at a community meeting at my first Summer Workshop, he stood up and proclaimed that he'd had heart surgery a few months before. He went on to say that he felt that the problem had been that his heart hadn't been open enough, and that he was going to work on opening it.

I took my problem to Sol, anticipating his ear and his wise counsel. What I didn't anticipate was the gift he gave me. After I told him my situation, he took my arm and steered us to an empty room, where he revealed an intimate, extremely personal, and very vulnerable piece of information about himself that bore directly on my issue, and implied guidance in the tenderest way possible. I've carried that scene deep inside myself ever since.

Finally, my longest standing mentor relationship in the Academy is with my family group. I can't say enough about the way the members have held me, confronted me, and influenced the way I've practiced psychotherapy. I've had the great good fortune to have spent many hours over a more than 40-year span in the company of courageous, caring and sensitive people who also happen to be gifted therapists. I've watched them struggle with life issues and be with each other, and with me, in growth-affirming ways that have stretched me as a person and taught me about being a therapist and a person in ways both describable and far beyond words.

In these last decades of my career, I have had the opportunity to teach, train, supervise and mentor a number of younger colleagues. Teaching in some way has always been in my mix of professional activities. I enjoy it, and it's felt a part of my drive to give back some of what I've been given. The more recent past has seen a shift from classroom teaching (dreams, group therapy) to individual and group supervision. I feel the presence of my mentors as I sit with my supervisees. I'm touched to watch as young therapists become less extensions of what should be done (in accordance with some real or imagined set of rules) and more trusting of their inner resources. I feel that much that I was given through contact with my mentors I've taken in and is now a part of my cell structure, although I do hear particular pieces of counsel in the remembered voices of particular mentors.

I feel that much of what I've tried to pass along rippled from the wisdom passed to me in encounters such as those I've recounted. The Academy has been the container for experiences that have shaped the person and therapist I am. I was in a group with Alex Redmountain and, at one point, said that I was feeling stupid. Alex said that "stupid" wasn't on the list of adjectives that he'd apply to me, but that my problem was that I didn't listen to my own voice. I remember not understanding what he'd meant. That evening I was in an intense conversation with another member, and, with an awareness I'd never experienced before, I heard myself. It was just as Alex had said, and I found myself able to respond from a place of new self-awareness. I feel grateful to the Academy and to its members who have given me so much. I honor them in my efforts to transmit what I have learned. I feel humbled to see myself as another link.

Elizabeth, a brilliant young psychologist that I've been supervising for a number of years, works with a caseload of very challenging people who constantly push her limits and require flexibility, spontaneity and humanity. She talks with trepidation about an exchange with a patient who's both fragile and anxious, and asks me how much I think she should reveal about her reactions to her. The words of one of my dear former therapists come to mind, and I tell her about it. He said to me, "You can say whatever comes to mind, as long as you remember who you are and what you're there for. Who you are is the therapist, and what you're there for is the growth and repair of the patient." I watch her relief as I tell her about this meaningful experience of mine and pass to her words that I've found useful and that have held me.

And so, it goes.

Commentary

"In every heart there is a room
A sanctuary safe and strong
To heal the wounds from lovers past
Until a new one comes along"
—(Billy Joel, "And So it Goes")

Barry's piece, and the final note on which he leaves us, reminded me of the Billy Joel song *"And So It Goes,"* which begins with the line, *"In every heart, there is a room / A sanctuary safe and strong."* It made me think of the rooms (and hearts) that have led me to become the therapist I am now—and how many of those sanctuaries were discovered through my AAP connections.

I appreciate getting to know Barry through the lens of a brand-new therapist, yearning for a professional home that matched what he believed good therapy ought to be: relational, personal, and human. As he takes us through the different moments that led him to become both a member and a leader in the organization, he shows how his willingness to be authentic and true to himself allowed him to enjoy and be enriched by meaningful connections with AAP members across generations.

So many of us who come to AAP through mentors, colleagues, or friends find ourselves, like Barry, in similar rooms—having deep conversations about what truly "works" in therapy, and how to remain human, and to sometimes struggle, while being a therapist. We also gain the chance to experience *what works* firsthand, and to witness how an intergenerational professional community can help heal the wounds of our relational pasts. Even before reading about how meaningful it is for Barry to be a link in the chain of giving and receiving shared knowledge, I already knew it to be true from every interaction I've had with him. Warm, generous, and spontaneous, Barry always offers golden moments that remain with me—moments I expect to pass on myself one day.

Barry's journey—from his earliest mentorship to the wisdom he now imparts to his supervisees—reminds us that the path of becoming a therapist is lifelong, full of personal discovery, risks, and opportunities. Ultimately, Barry's story offers a relational lesson: we find strength, wisdom, and courage in what we pass from person to person.

—Abby MacDonald, LCSW

Commentary

THIS PIECE IS A MARVELOUS DETAILED RECOUNTING OF THE AUTHOR'S PRIMARY INFLUENCES AS A PSYCHOTHERAPIST, INCLUDING SEVERAL IMPORTANT PEOPLE IN AAP HISTORY. A mother who was caring and sensitive can be added to this list, a foundation for the author's sensibilities about what feels right in early attempts to find a psychology that fits. I really like how the author parses out various training experiences, gradually getting closer, some of them "still off the mark," trying them on until something else fits better with who they are and how they want to practice.

For me, the message here is the key to why AAP can be so transformative—the power of sharing personal, vulnerable experiences with other trusted therapists who help us repair and become freer to grow, and then to be able to "pass it on" to future generations.

There is a lovely full-circle feeling, from the author's early attempts to trust inner knowing, to the reminder from Alex Redmountain to "listen to your own voice." I appreciate the example at the end of how the author remembers the words of a former therapist while working with a supervisee. What a beautiful tribute that is. A paraphrase of that quote would be frameable: "Remember who you are and that you're there for the growth and repair of the patient."

—Peggy Brooks, PhD

Be patient toward all that is unsolved in
your heart and try to love the questions
themselves, like locked rooms and like books
that are now written in a very foreign tongue.

Do not seek the answers, which cannot be given
you because you would not be able to live them.
And the point is, to live everything.

Live the questions now. Perhaps you will then
gradually, without noticing it, live along
some distant day into the answer.
—Ranier Maria Rilke

Jonathan Farber

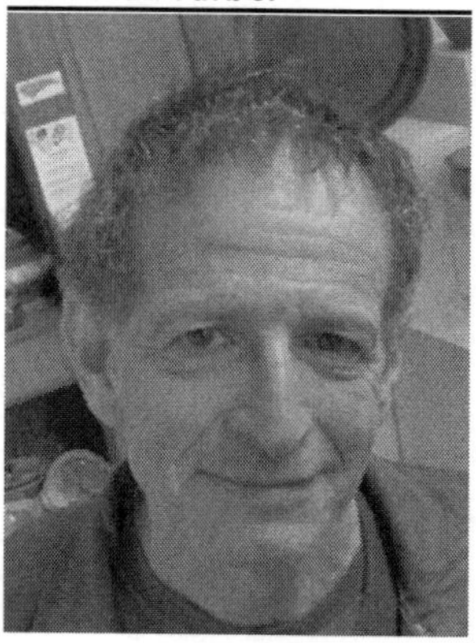

JONATHAN FARBER PHD is a clinical psychologist who practices in Washington DC and Chapel Hill, NC, providing individual and group psychotherapy and supervision. He has received extensive training from his children and his border collie, as well as from his teachers at Duke University, his patients, and his colleagues in AAP. He and Tom Burns edited *Voices* from 2003–2009.

Questions and Contradictions: Mentoring and the Psychotherapy Relationship

Who knows the most?
The person who can learn from anyone.
—The Talmud

MOST OF US WOULD AGREE THAT THE PRODUCTIVE EXPERIENCES PATIENTS HAVE IN PSYCHOTHERAPY CANNOT BE SEPARATED FROM THE RELATIONSHIP WITH THE THERAPIST. Likewise, I cannot separate the lessons I have learned about how to practice psychotherapy from the relationships where I learned them. I've had wonderful experiences being mentored in the practice of psychotherapy, as well as meaningful experiences mentoring other therapists, and over the years I learned still more in the relationships I've had with my clients. That's a lot of lessons, from a lot of sources, and I do have some good days, when it seems as if all the pieces have stitched themselves together into the intricate and beautiful quilt of my professional identity, my personal style of doing "the work." Other days, I think it's still a mess, a cacophony of voices interrupting and contradicting each other. Here are some of the separate pieces. See if they cohere for you.

My first clinical supervisor, Lloyd Borstelmann, had spent a lifetime working with children and their families, and we couldn't have been more different. I had always been a serious kid, and a serious student, and while at Duke I was constantly afraid I'd make some goof that would get me thrown out of the program and barred from the career I wanted so badly. I could get animated and occasionally fierce in class discussions, but mostly I

> [Lloyd] always encouraged me to be creative about the form and organization of the therapy, and was excited when I improvised with structure and boundaries. "Respect for the client," he would repeat to me. "Everything else is negotiable, as long as we have respect for the client."

tried to camouflage myself in jeans and faded flannel. Lloyd was quite a showman—an amateur actor who often performed in local theater—who showed me how much of therapy is showmanship, not for ego, but for communication and impact. He was playful, and readily amused, and somehow, he usually got us both laughing during supervision. Whenever he told me "We must listen, really listen, to the client, he'd cup his hand theatrically behind his ear." The first couple I worked with had intense fights, and each time I brought that case into supervision, Lloyd would shadowbox briefly, showing me that the fights were also drama: ritualized, and potentially quite funny.

Unashamed of his occasional memory lapses— "Refresh my memory, wouldja?"—and unashamed to fart audibly, he didn't mock or embarrass me for my seriousness, which would have been so easy to do. He just shared himself and his thoughts about my clients and what I was doing with them, as his joyfulness and relaxed attitude about psychotherapy gradually percolated into me.

In my final session with that couple, Lloyd's lessons paid off when I decided to address one of their remaining areas of friction, the wife's complaint that the husband—of course he was named Rod—wanted sex even at unsuitable times. Judiciously, thinking to explore the subtleties of their communication, I asked her what, for instance, made her think he wanted sex last night? "Well, he was standing there with his dick in his hands, waving it at me," she laughed. "Do you think I was jumping to conclusions?" I looked over at him, and for an instant he looked a little embarrassed, but then he tipped his head to one side, shrugged, and started laughing too. I knew I had been their straight man in the joke, but when I released my formal pretenses, abandoned my plan for the session, and allowed my own laughter to slip out, I could see that my concern and respect for them had registered, and that I was temporarily included in the warmth and love that hummed beneath the surface of their arguments.

When Lloyd was widowed, I ached for him; a couple years later, beaming, he announced his engagement and invited me to his outdoor wedding, adding that he was particularly pleased that "she is a lady of my own vintage."

He always encouraged me to be creative about the form and organization of the therapy, and was excited when I improvised with structure and boundaries. "Respect for the client," he would repeat to me. "Everything else is negotiable, as long as we have respect for the client," and he would listen carefully (and respectfully) to my rationale for whatever I was proposing to do clinically. I hear his voice again whenever I am considering doing something unconventional in therapy, or when I want to understand my negative reactions to a client. Do I respect them? Does my respect show? I can still see dapper Lloyd dressed all in gleaming white for his wedding under the pergola in Duke Gardens, from his white fedora to his white loafers, save for the piercing blue cornflower in his lapel: a cheerful old man at ease under the bright lights on center stage.

An AAP conference once opened with the metaphor of a quilt representing the Academy, and everyone attending was invited to announce who in the Academy had been a trusted mentor, and their names were somehow attached to a quilt on the front wall. I may have been the only one in room both engaged enough and detached enough to be counting, but by my count Alex Redmountain was the mentor named by the greatest number. This helped me override my habitual mistrust of authority, and eventually I managed to nudge myself into his orbit by signing up for a workshop he was leading where he influenced me more than he could have known with a brief remark. I was on a roll, sharing my reactions to the other members, and he had already complimented me on my analyses of the group's dynamics. A little intoxicated from the praise, I took a wilder leap and simply guessed at something I thought one woman was feeling, and it landed well, unlocking a surge of emotion from her. Alex said: "You're not only very thoughtful, you're also quite intuitive." Unstinting affirmation like that wasn't something I had known even existed. It changed the way I saw myself, helped me grow more self-confident, and ultimately enabled me to pass along that level of affirmation to others. Intuition in particular wasn't something I'd ever aspired to, nor thought I possessed. Alex's comment showed me the power that something as simple as authentic affirmation can have in a relationship, and his specific affirmation also made me realize that as a therapist I had been wasting a lot of words explaining and justifying my perceptions. I discovered that in the context of a trusting relationship with me, patients could usually just take my unadorned perceptions and run with them. Me, always the hyper-rational one, now an intuitive: who knew?

Over many years I've learned to listen differently to the answers to my questions, listening for what's beneath the spoken answers—the emotion, the transference, the assumptions about causality, about relationships—and decades after Lloyd's death, I realized with a wince that when he was telling me to listen to patients, I had been too busy searching his words for more arcane and mysterious techniques to really listen to him. I'm not sure, years later, that I could process all the complexity that I used to think about so busily in the course of a therapy session, but I don't seem to need to: my intuitive or holistic grasp of the client's predicament is simpler, as are my interventions. It is as if my unconscious is reducing fractions before they even become conscious—why think 17/51 when you can think one third? I'd like to think that this means I'm tracking it all at a deeper level. I don't hear myself speak as many words now, either. I'd like to think that's because I'm clearer about what I want to say before I begin speaking.

"It is as if my unconscious is reducing fractions before they even become conscious—why think 17/51 when you can think one third?"

"Less judgment, more curiosity" was a lesson Alex had for everyone, patients and therapists alike, and it has become something of an Academy anthem. But it was only in my relationships with patients that I came to my own understanding of the phrase. Judgment is anger that is afraid to show itself directly: shaming to the recipient, and unsatisfying to the angry one posing as a neutral judge.

And how can I list the many lessons my clients have taught me? I should say at the outset here that I accomplish most of my work by asking questions. I find questions to be a gentle and respectful way of guiding attention: attention to what has been overlooked, yearned for, forgotten, or feared. When I ask questions instead of delivering pronouncements or prescriptions, we can both learn. Besides, my patients' real lives and their internet lives are both full of people who have so much to tell them. What is special—and potentially transformative—is someone who wants to listen to them.

In my early years as a therapist, I thought that if I asked a question, for instance about a feeling or a memory, and the client didn't know the answer, then the entire interaction was a Fail: awkward and a waste of precious session time, and an embarrassing demonstration that I wasn't really tracking the client as well as I should. But now I often find myself re-asking the same unanswered questions, because clients often eventually do answer the question (on the second try, or the tenth). Ultimately, I learned that an unanswered question is not necessarily a Fail at all. When we work a pump handle at a well, the water column in the pipe, invisible in the bedrock under our feet, rises a little closer to the surface with each repetition. Seeking inside oneself can bring one closer to an answer in ways that are not visible until the fifth or tenth iteration, when the answer breaks the surface.

"Seeking inside oneself can bring one closer to an answer in ways that are not visible until the fifth or tenth iteration, when the answer breaks the surface."

One of my first patients, a recovering anorexic, a timid veteran of many therapy relationships herself, taught me to speak regular English, rather than the Psychology Speak I'd learned in graduate school. She noticed immediately when I sometimes dropped the formalities, and she felt more comfortable with that version of me: "Just be yourself Jon, be someone who can relate to me." It was great advice. I could see how much less self-conscious she became, how much more capable of reflection and change, when I talked to her, my client, the way I would talk to a person. I could see that when I had the courage to be more myself, it helped her to do likewise. So what if this was her idea and not mine—it was still a good idea.

Some of my early professors were enamored of the family systems model, one of the great therapy fads of the 80s. As I read the literature, the clinical application of this model always seemed to hold the parents responsible for the family's "enmeshment:" the child's inadequacies and dependency were blamed on the parents over functioning and clinginess. But when I listened to the parents in families I worked with, I often heard a convincing account of a child with a long history of needing extra help. The protracted parental oversight was a caring response to the child's struggles, not its cause. I had been taught that most psychopathology begins with bad parenting, but my work with patients exposed me to many wonderful parents who raised struggling and suffering children, as well as to many abysmal parents whose children thrived. Since then, of

"When I began my practice, I was very clear that I didn't want to become a famous psychologist, because… I didn't want to hear myself reciting the same speeches again and again."

course, family systems theory has had its hour (OK, maybe seven years) in the spotlight, and faded. By now I've seen so many models and theories and Three-or-Four-First-Initial-Therapies (TOFFITs) come and go that it's difficult for me to take any of them too seriously. I do generally have a model or map in my head of what we are working on in therapy, but I try to derive these afresh from what I see of each particular client, rather than leading with some model and then finding a place in it where the client can be installed.

In the first years of my practice, I tried to continue seeing clients who thought their therapy was complete, if I did not agree that it was, and I tried to terminate clients whom I thought were finished, even if they thought we should continue. The ones I prevailed on to continue didn't accomplish much more. The ones who stayed in therapy despite my recommendation to terminate consistently achieved new levels of insight and change. So collectively they taught me something I can summarize in a few admittedly controversial words: people know what they need.

When I began my practice, I was very clear that I didn't want to become a famous psychologist, because of two things I didn't want in my life. I didn't want to spend a lot of nights in hotel rooms, away from my family (this was before the internet enabled us to reach a national audience without traveling) and I didn't want to hear myself reciting the same speeches again and again. What keeps work engaging for me is the unexpected things my clients have to say, and the varied and often novel tacks I have to come up with to be helpful. Famous psychologists become famous by honing and repeating their own messages endlessly.

Nevertheless, when I was recently invited to be the headliner at a small conference, I felt a little differently. After 44 years of continuous practice, I do have things I want to teach. In AAP, I like that we take turns being the teacher to each other. Some of us take on the teacher role only after decades in the student role, when our own teachers have passed from the scene. Others feel like we do enough "teaching" in our clinical work, and take on only the student role at conferences. Sometimes we choose to play both roles, at different workshops within a single conference. To me, AAP's structure is the opposite of what I encountered in my internship at a Duke Medical Center, where the rigid hierarchy in the staff, between supervisors and providers, was mirrored in the relationship between providers and patients. That is where I discovered on my own how easy it is to make patients intimidated and compliant, and how much more challenging and worthwhile it is to enable them to feel safe, respected, and empowered.

Here's one more thought about the teacher-student relationship, from someone

"A student can learn without a teacher—much of what I know I learned on my own. But a teacher can't teach without a student: the greater debt of gratitude—though it's not often acknowledged—is owed by the teacher."

who's been both. A student can learn without a teacher—much of what I know I learned on my own. But a teacher can't teach without a student: the greater debt of gratitude—though it's not often acknowledged—is owed by the teacher.

Psychotherapy is most fundamentally a relationship between two unique people, which is why I find psychotherapy difficult to teach or even describe didactically. The most valuable training I have received or given has always been in the context of a teaching relationship. These relationships are sometimes labeled (way too simplistically) clinical supervision, or sometimes (less hierarchically) clinical consultation. In a teaching relationship, as in therapy, we can begin with questions about repeated patterns and combinations of, say, bodily sensations, interpersonal behavior, thoughts and emotions. Student therapists can lean in and feel what their own patients experience as they struggle towards deeper self-awareness, and also how complex, vulnerable, and emotionally intense it can be to receive and accept help. In a teaching relationship, the student therapists can step back and observe the patterns in themselves that play out in all their relationships, including when they are the therapist. As the teacher, I can demonstrate with the student therapist the process of tracking the client's experience so very closely that as each answer raises further questions, I can gradually get the feel for the person: their map of the world and how it operates, their self-image, their vocabulary, and the embedded rhythm and inflections of their speech. It's like internalizing a working model of the person: useful for whatever change we undertake.

As in any intimate relationship, the ego boundaries between teacher and student grow porous, and ideas for intentional change the student therapist might seek, or that I might propose, encourage, coax, or invite, are experienced as originating from "us" rather than from either of us separately. My enthusiasm and confidence are sustained by my certainty that there are no wrong turns when we risk initiating a change: even if it doesn't work as we'd hoped, we will learn from whatever happens. (You, the reader, may like this article so far, or you may not—either way, together we can explore the reasons for your reactions, and see what we learn).

More questions will lead us to more pieces of the puzzle, some of which may contradict others—but that's great, because contradictions offer another great entry into deeper inquiry. Contradictions intrigue us, and invite us to seek out the overlooked, repressed, and banished parts of the self, and spur us to find ways to integrate them. "You handle criticism at work so much better than you do at home—why is that?" Or, "Those two members of your therapy group complain about such similar problems, but you feel compassion for this one yet judgment towards that one—why is that?"

When my patients or my students allow me to see them struggle for so long on fundamental issues—coping with emotions, loss, pain, social self-image and identity—they are teaching me that they can lose heart and momentum, and that what they need from me is to direct their attention (yes, often using questions) to the progress they've already made, so that we can affirm it, celebrate it, and hopefully expand on it. "You are handling criticism at work so much better than you used to: that's your new template. Now you're trying to figure out how to do that at home." Supporting their morale when they are heading in the right direction, so that they don't give up too soon, is not a showy role for me to play—it's not centerstage—but I have other places in my life where those needs for the spotlight and attention are met: at work I find that I am satisfied to earn nothing more than a "best supporting actor" award.

My patients who needed (and deserved) apologies from me taught me that I don't lose any gravitas by apologizing. In fact, I think I gain respect as well as trust when I do. And speaking of mistakes, one of my mentors, an ethics mavin, once said in a workshop: "When the therapist disappoints the client—really, seriously lets them down—that's when the therapy starts." I return to that line again and again when therapy gets rough, and I start to doubt myself. "Of course you screwed up," I say, in a judo move on my inner critic, "and that's good, because this is where the relationship gets real." Whatever we work out from that point on will have more depth and meaning, and more applicability to their real-life relationships, because—not in spite of—the awkward and problematic moments between us, because once they surface, we can name and explore them.

To see another person as an individual takes patience—two or even ten data points are not enough to give you all your answers. Before you, for instance, is never just another patient on the autism spectrum with OCD features and mild depressive episodes, or another a politically leftwing white hetero female accountant. One has to keep asking for more, even when the person identifies strongly with a category, or presents it to me as if that's all I should need to know about them before I can tell them how to proceed in life. I like to work with their group identifications around two questions, presented with genuine curiosity: What do you have in common with all the other people in your category, and what distinguishes you from all the other people in your category i.e., how are you unique within that group? With answers to those questions on the table, we can look at what the identification with a particular category actually means to the person, and we can have conversations about the person as the particular individual they are, and not simply as the incarnation of an abstract identity class.

This is related to my personal aversion to "specialization" in psychotherapy. I do understand the attraction of specialization as a marketing tool, and as self-reassurance when a therapist feels anxious or stymied in the work of helping someone ("I'm the local expert in this condition, I teach CE courses in it, plus I've got my certification in my TOFFIT"). But if we truly believe in the uniqueness of the individual, then each person is in their own diagnostic category, and isn't specialization meaningless? I find that when I think of myself as a specialist in say, anxiety, I'm calling myself an expert in anxiety. I know what causes it, I know the "Six Leading Types" of it, I know the cures for it, and I begin to sound like a self-help video or an AI. I stop listening to the patient and am only listening to myself. Some of this inflated confidence may temporarily rub off on a patient who believes in me, but as with therapy based on the pursuit of emotional catharsis, the improvement doesn't last because the emotional dynamics inside the person haven't changed.

Also related is my preference for very long-term relationships in psychotherapy. I am fascinated by the long arcs in human development. To even perceive these in an individual, let alone shift them, is the work of years. Along the way, the therapist acquires a tremendous quantity of person-specific knowledge: one might say the therapist becomes a specialist in that particular individual. Yes, it is slow work, but for me the satisfaction of seeing that I've had an unmistakable and positive impact on the life of that unique individual is unequalled, a fulfillment that remains with me always.

As I said at the beginning, I believe that teaching the practice of therapy, like therapy itself, can only happen in the context of a living relationship, where the question and answer dynamic is bespoke and continuously emergent; it is an intimacy that temporarily transcends ego boundaries, and—as with parenting—it is an intimacy where one person can loan another some ego strength (emotional stability, self-esteem, and hope) until it becomes internalized. And yet, as I read the paragraphs above, I must acknowledge that in this piece I am plainly trying to reach an anonymous readership with whom I do not have an ongoing relationship, contradicting myself by trying to do what I said can't be done. I suspect that the approaching end of my career gives an urgency to my wish to pass on what I've learned, even if it means holding a contradiction to be worked out later, [sigh]. To resolve all our internal conflicts and integrate all our diverse pieces, I am now old enough to say with confidence, is the work of more than a lifetime, and speaking for myself, I don't expect to complete it. And in keeping with an article celebrating questions and contradictions, I should really conclude now with both—but how am I supposed to do that?

You cannot teach a man anything.

You can only help him discover it within himself.

—Galileo Galilei

Avrum G. Weiss

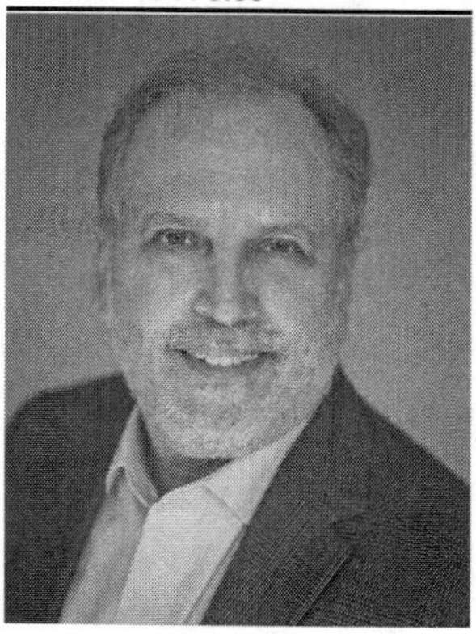

Avrum G. Weiss, PhD, is an author and psychotherapist. He is the author of four books, including the best-selling *Hidden in Plain Sight: How Men's Fears of Women Shape Their Intimate Relationships.* Avrum is also a regular contributor to psychologytoday.com He lives on an island in mid-coast Maine and also on a sailboat in the Bahamas.
agweiss1953@me.com

The Art of Psychotherapy and The Psychotherapy of Art

Introduction

The title of this journal is "Voices: The Art and Science of Psychotherapy." The phrase "Art of psychotherapy" began to be explicitly used in academic and popular discourse in the mid-20th century as many therapists challenged the extent to which psychotherapy could or should be conceptualized within the constraints of the natural sciences paradigm (Giorgi, 1970). Many psychotherapists (May, 1958; Perls, 1951; Rogers, 1951; Szasz, 1961; Whitaker, C. & Malone, T., 1981; Winnicott, 1965; Yalom, 1980) used the term "Art" in an attempt to capture the unique, irreducible relational aspects of each therapeutic encounter. Others in the field have a stronger allegiance to the scientific aspects of the work and believe that conceptualizing psychotherapy as an art detracts from its status as a science.

Anecdotally, many psychotherapists are also drawn to parallel work as artists in various forms of expression. For some of these therapists, art is more of a hobby, something they do for pleasure; for others, their work as artists is a second career, and they identify as much as artists as they do as psychotherapists. Drs. Fern Beu and David Pellegrini are two such therapists, both of whom have had substantial careers and recognition as artists that rival their decades of practice as senior clinicians. They are also dear friends and colleagues who have inspired each other on their journeys to become artists.

This article is based on interviews with these remarkable professionals who stand at the intersection of art and psychotherapy and have much to teach us about how each discipline can inform and elevate the other.

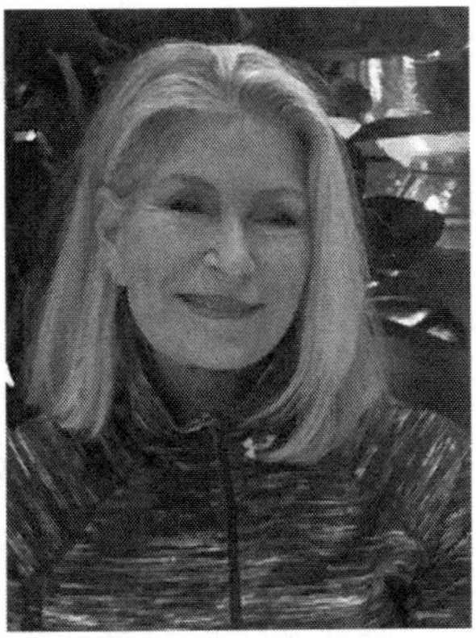

FERN BEU, PHD, has been in private practice in Washington DC and Maryland since 1980. In addition to running groups, and seeing individuals and couples, a substantial part of her practice is supervising other therapists in their private practices. She began her life as a painter in 1951 with a watercolor class and has been devoted to becoming a better artist ever since. She is a portrait and figurative artist primarily, and enjoys painting animals. She has had many solo shows and is included in the Governor's book of prominent Maryland artists, and was featured in an Eastern shore magazine lead article. She is grateful to have the two best jobs in the world! *fbeau@icloud.com*

Their work, whether expressed through painting, photography, writing, or therapeutic dialogue, reveals a profound commitment to understanding the complexity of the human experience through scientific inquiry and creative expression. Their journeys reveal that the deep, reflective processes involved in psychotherapy inform their creative practices and, in turn, their art enhances the more creative aspects of their therapeutic work. Such a synthesis offers a fresh perspective on both domains, illustrating that in the nuanced world of human experience, art and psychotherapy are not merely separate pursuits but are mutually transformative.

Therapeutic and Artistic Histories.

Fern and David started from different backgrounds regarding their art, yet they have come to similar places. Fern's lifelong relationship with art began in childhood. As she recalls, *"I never had dolls. I had easels, tempera, and pencils. I was responsive to color from a very young age, and (some of) my earliest memories are of going to museums. My mother desperately wanted me to be an artist."* Fern put her work as a visual artist aside during graduate school because she grew up in a family that lost all of their money and did not believe she could make a reliable living as an artist, but she never lost her passionate connection to the art world. Twenty-five years ago, she began her work as a painter.

Twenty-five years ago, she began her work as a painter. Once she started, Fer was surprised by the level of passion she experienced, which has continued unabated, *"obsessional in the best possible way." Fern added, "I have been so fortunate that David and I have—this makes me want to cry, sorry—have this partnership. David and I have put ourselves out in ways that I normally would never have put myself out in order to passionately go after something that we both adore and that has fulfilled us in different ways."*

David's artistic narrative is equally compelling but emerged from his unique familial and personal pressures. He, also, recognized his interest in the arts as a young child, but, unlike in Fern's family, his father's practical bent and emphasis on financial security tempered his interest in pursuing life as an artist. David said, *"My father was the hardest working man I ever knew, (he was) from an immigrant family, and what he saw as his responsibility was to lift everyone up out of poverty. I was supposed to do something that would pay well. I was supposed to be anything but an artist."* A childhood illness, however, catalyzed David's creative yearning. He got sick with rheumatic fever in the eighth

DAVID PELLEGRINI, PHD, is a clinical psychologist in private practice in Washington, DC. Previously, he was a tenured Associate Professor of Psychology at The Catholic University of America. In addition to psychotherapy, he provides consultation to businesses on leadership and succession planning. He is also an avid representational oil painter, fine art photographer, and writer. His pursuit of artistic development provides considerable joy and meaning to his life, along with endless challenges. Self portrait by David Pellegrini. *dspellegini@gmail.com*

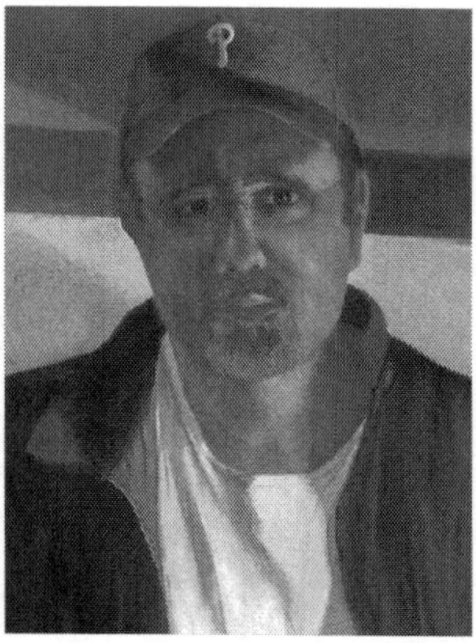

grade and missed almost the entire school year. David had two older cousins who were high school teachers who *"started feeding me stimulation. They (would) arrive at my bedside with these art books and they (would) come over and watch foreign films with me, and it was like my head exploded. I felt like I have got to tap into that vein of creative expression, and I found myself looking around for some way to do that. So, I took a summer class in printmaking. I started writing. I was writing poetry and short stories and anything I could do to express some of my passionate, emotional feelings."* A mentor encouraged David to express his creativity by studying psychology. *"I kind of put down my interest in painting…I was intimidated. I felt more capable as a writer than in painting or drawing, and so I put it down. I became a psychotherapist but it wasn't all of what I had inside of me, and something felt missing. That longing for something that was more creative, self-expression, for making something new, for doing something that was uniquely me. Really, until I came across Fern pursuing her class work, and I said to myself, 'What am I doing? I've always wanted to do this. Why am I not doing it?' It's like I borrowed courage from her to go after a process that I wanted to engage in and that literally changed my life."*

Timing.

David and Fern both came to their work as artists in the second half of their lives and both plan to continue their careers as artists after ending their careers as psychotherapists. I asked if they had begun their careers as artists, might they have found that path satisfying and not pursued careers as psychotherapists? David answered, *"I can't imagine not having been a psychotherapist. It's been a remarkably enriching life, and I really do think being a therapist for me has made my art better. When I look back on my life, I don't think I would want to make my living just as an artist because I feel like I'm doing it much more for myself."*

Fern added, "There's no way I could have ever been successful as an artist had I not become a psychotherapist and had my own therapy first, because my character problems would have destroyed my capacity to experiment (and to) know when I was getting in my own way."

Is everyone creative?

I asked Fern and David if they believe that everyone is creative and has the desire or perhaps even the need to express themselves in some creative fashion. Fern pointed out that *"The drive to make art goes back to the cave paintings. There's kind of an innate (drive) to create something outside of themselves that has harmony or beauty."* David agreed, saying that *"Everybody has creativity in them, everyone has something to say, (whether) they choose to express it (which is) not to say that everybody has (the) natural born talent to draw ... (or) have a certain eye... but you don't need that to be an artist."*

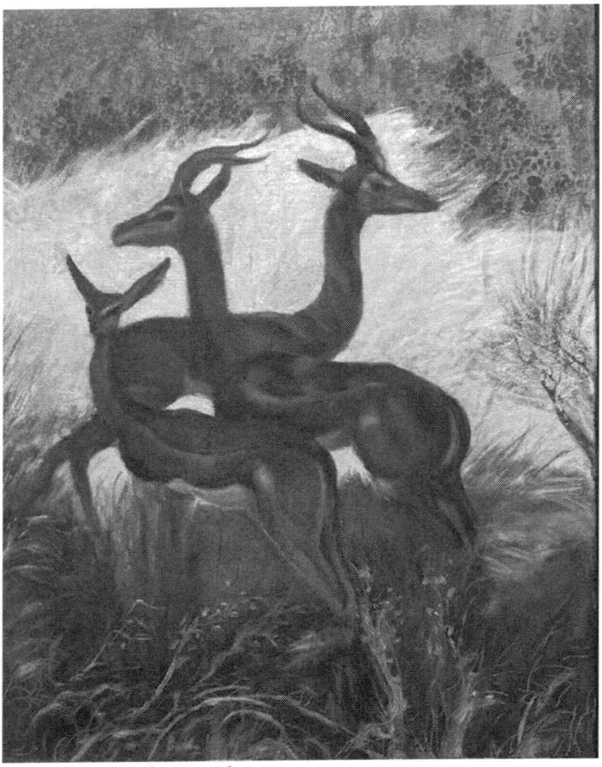

African Antelopes by Fern Bleu

Does everyone need to create?

David and Fern both believe that honoring their creativity and finding ways to express it and develop it has been an essential part of their lives. They have also each had significant periods in their lives in which they were not making art. So, I asked them what it was like when they were not honoring and developing their creativity and whether they believed that developing one's creative potential was an essential aspect of a good life. David said, *"When I have had dry periods of making art, whether it's writing or painting or Photography, when it's fallen by the wayside because I've been too busy, I am acutely aware of feeling a little depressed, feeling like I'm not right, I'm not me."* This creative deprivation translates into a sense of disconnection not only from his artistic identity but also from his capacity as a therapist. By returning to art, David reconnects with the core of who he is, infusing his therapeutic practice with renewed energy and insight. In contrast, Fern maintained a connection with her creativity during the first part of her life when she was not actively engaged in making art. *"I guess I didn't feel like I was missing it because I was still going to museums and still interested in art."*

Talent is a double-edged sword.

I was intrigued by David's statement that talent is not necessary to create art, so I asked what role talent has in artistic creation. David said he was *"Born with kind of an artistic temperament in how I view the world, I was always looking at things visually,"* but he never thought of himself as having "natural" talent." He believes that he became a good artist in the same way he became a psychotherapist, through a determination to master a set of skills. David said, *"My sense or my belief or judgment that I had to have innate talent held me back for a long, long time, maybe half my life."* Fern said, *"It's about our joint desire to be the best, to do whatever it takes, (this) need to get to a level of excellence is embedded in my deep desire to be taken seriously, to be seen and to be respected... I finally realized why I never did it, despite the fact of always thinking I'm going to do it, and that was because I wouldn't be good, and as long as I didn't actually try it, I could hold on to the fantasy that someday I'd be good."* David added, *"Knowing what's good and what's great has driven both of us in our psychotherapy practice, and it's driven both of us in our artistic practice, and we've both been exposed to people who are outstanding in both domains, so the standards that we each set are high."* Fern described the crippling despair that can arise when she feels incapable of producing art that meets her high standards, which she equates to the self-doubt many therapists experience, especially in the early years of practice.

David reflected on the terror he sometimes experiences when beginning a new painting, and both agreed that the therapeutic environment can offer a structure that can buffer against overwhelming self-criticism. Both practitioners have, over time, learned to view self-judgment as a natural, if painful, component of their creative and clinical work. David finds that the very process of struggling through creative despair can yield work that is both deeply personal and resonant. This willingness to engage with vulnerability ultimately propels them forward in both domains.

For Fern, the validation from sharing her art, especially when her work is purchased by someone who truly connects with its narrative, is a critical hedge against her inner critic. She said, *"I've always wanted to, not just be a good artist, but also to have artistic success."* Selling his work is a different experience for David. *"I have a certain feeling like I'm giving away a part of myself when I sell my favorite paintings."* Fern responded: *"I always sell my best paintings. It helps me if I sell them to someone I know because I can imagine them in their home, and I have a warm feeling of the connection. But when I sell one of them to somebody I don't know, (I) never stop thinking about those paintings."*

The Influence of Clinical Practice and Personal Psychotherapy on Artistic Practice.

Both Fern and David began their professional careers as psychologists, and their work as professional artists came later in their careers. One of the premises of this article is that the influence of these two endeavors on each other is reciprocal, that is to say, that training and experience as a psychotherapist influence practice as an artist, just as practice as an artist also influences work as a psychotherapist. Beginning one's career as an artist and then training as a psychotherapist would undoubtedly result in a different story unfolding. Still, the relationship between the two would remain reciprocal.

Practicing as a psychotherapist offers endless opportunities for developing a profound and intimate understanding of one's character. For depth psychotherapists, the individual character of the psychotherapist is inevitably and necessarily revealed in and plays an essential role in the practice of psychotherapy. For Fern and David, the same is true in their artistic work. Fern said that every character flaw she has worked on in

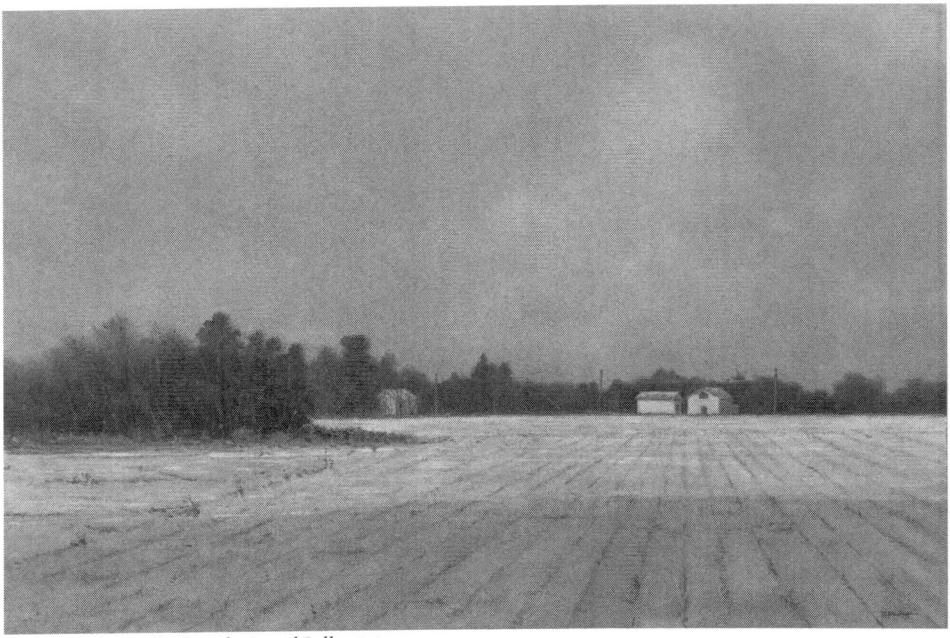

Winter Settles on the Farm by David Pellegrini

therapy also emerges in her work as an artist, and that she could not have become as successful as an artist without her experience as both a patient and a therapist. Mentors who helped Fern understand how those characterological issues impacted her work have been an essential part of her development as an artist.

There are, of course, therapists who think of the therapist's characterological issues as impediments that should be excluded from the therapeutic relationship, just as there are artists who work to exclude their person from their work as artists. Fern equated psychotherapy without an intimate relationship to being rigidly committed to painting in a certain style. Fern describes this art as lacking in "value, shifts, and depth," comparing it to manualized psychotherapy. Fern said *"It's so clear to me my whole process and how I work with a person before I actually do their portrait comes directly out of my training as a psychotherapist."* Fern said that whenever she paints a portrait, she *"falls in love with that person, seeing in them a tapestry of vulnerabilities and strengths that would be impossible to capture with a mere technical exercise."* She added, *"They become an object of beauty to me."* For Fern, there are parallels in her work as a psychotherapist. *"When I take somebody (in)to therapy, as I really look at them, really see them, and I see their parts and how they interact and how they don't interact, and when they, you know, clash with connection, or clash with me, or diminish a person, they become beautiful to me. And I think that quality of absorbing myself into who they are in a way that wants to bring forth beauty, is one of the things that makes me a good psychotherapist."*

Similarly, David's work in portrait photography, most notably an evocative project in Cuba, is marked by an intensive process of engaging with his subjects long before capturing their image, a process he learned in his work as a psychotherapist to use deep listening and a genuine interest in another's inner world to guide the creative process. He said he *"spent hours with those people that I photographed, hours and hours and hours talking to them with a translator, most of the time, hearing their life story, finding something out about them before I ever put them in a pose or context."* David believes he could not have done this work without his training as a psychotherapist and experience as a patient. *"I wouldn't have known how, or have even known that was something you could do, because your vision is with another person or your encounter with the landscape, (then) what you end up producing, hopefully, is a reflection of you in relation to your subject matter."*

Mastery in both fields also requires letting go of reliance on techniques to bring more of oneself to an inherently intimate encounter. Dick Felder compared this to the process of a jazz musician learning how to improvise, pointing out that each musician needed to first learn the appropriate musical techniques to play music and then forget them to improvise (Felder &Weiss, 1991). Fern said, *"I thought, when I started, if I could just paint how something looked, then I'd become an artist. To my horror, I finally got good enough to copy things accurately most times, and it was so deflating. I got (to) that place where I could copy whatever, but then I didn't know what to paint because I wasn't moved. So how many times can you put a still life up and paint it? But what happened was I started having the themes that I was interested in, like my first solo show that I did was based on the life (of a woman) with whom I had a very special relationship (and) I adored."*

The Influence of Artistic Training on Clinical Practice.

Just as personal psychotherapy and professional practice enrich artistic expression, the creative process has a profound influence on the practice of therapy. Both Fern and David subscribe to one of the guiding principles of experiential psychotherapy, which is that it is the therapist's capacity for experience that sets the ceiling for the work the patient can do in psychotherapy (Felder & Weiss, 1991). They both believe that art is a vital means of self-exploration that allows them to access aspects of their character that might otherwise remain unknown and unavailable in their therapeutic relationships.

For example, one of David's early painting teachers pointed out the colors on his palette that he was overlooking- no red. She encouraged David to find the influence of red in the landscape he was painting, which David understood as an invitation to explore disowned aspects of himself. He's learned to apply the same process as a psychotherapist to help his patients wonder what "colors" they are missing in their lives and how they might find and utilize them more fully.

Fern described being the victim of familial violence as a child and learning strategies to protect herself from the emotional impact of that violence internally. Fern believes that the work she has done as an artist in learning to access the colors she had avoided has helped her work as a therapist in learning how to lean into people's unregulated affect rather than fleeing. David concurred, saying that as a therapist, he frequently thinks about his vision of the person he is working with. *"What do I see that maybe they don't see, their shadow or their potential, their ways of getting themselves into trouble, what they could become, where they might want to look."*

David and Fern emphasized the importance of how their work as artists has helped them learn to see the world in a different light. Fern said, *"I see things now instead of just looking at things. I see patterns, I see conversations between different elements. I see beauty in how colors harmonize with one another."* David added that there are times he has to be *"Careful I don't drive off the road sometimes, because there are moments (where I see) little jewels of light over a field or coming through (the) trees that just take your breath away ...(and) then it's gone... that ephemeral moment."* He drew a parallel to his work with patients, saying, *"I think a lot of patients that I've worked with, they miss those little jewels (in) their own lives . . . I'm very interested in the notion of re-enchantment with life, with aliveness, for people who are kind of depressed or anxious or living in the weeds to kind of get them to look around and pay attention."*

David and Fern also agreed they had learned much about timing and pacing in psychotherapy from their work as artists. David said that as a therapist, he is sometimes *"so eager to get to the good bits, the discoveries, that we get off to a (fast) start, and then it becomes hard to do the pick-and-shovel work of psychotherapy... Sometimes you have to go really slow to not get ahead of the patient in their journey. Like with painting, in building a picture you have to know what to leave out and what to add in."* He remembers Ray Lovett's saying that nothing does more damage to a patient than the therapist's need to be brilliant and how important it is to hold back and not insert yourself into any space the patient might expand into.

Conclusion.

Traditional models of therapy have been critiqued for their overemphasis on manualized techniques, which can render the therapeutic process formulaic and impersonal. In contrast, Fern and David represent a growing movement that views the "art" of therapy as an essential counterbalance to its scientific underpinnings. Both fields demand rigor and technical skill, yet both also require an intuitive, creative engagement with the human condition. The artful therapist is not merely a technician, but also, hopefully, a visionary who continually adapts and responds to the uniqueness of each encounter. In this way, art and psychotherapy are not opposed, but complement one another, each informing the other with new insights and modes of expression.

References:

Felder, R. & Weiss, A. (1991). Experiential Psychotherapy: A Symphony of Selves. University Press of America.

Giorgi, A. (1970). Psychology as a human science: A phenomenologically based approach.

Harper & Row

May, R. (1958). The Art of Counseling. Abingdon Press.

Perls, F. S., Hefferline, R., & Goodman, P. (1951). Gestalt Therapy: Excitement and Growth in the Human Personality.Julian Press.

Rogers, C. R. (1951). Client-Centered Therapy: Its Current Practice, Implications, and

Theory. Houghton Mifflin.

Szasz, T. (1961). The Myth of Mental Illness: Foundations of a Theory of Personal

Conduct. Harper & Row.

Weiss, A.G. (2011) Change Happens: When to Try Harder, and When to Stop Trying So Hard.

University Press of America.

Whitaker, C. & Malone, T. (1981). The Roots of Psychotherapy. Routledge.

Winnicott, D. W. (1965). The Maturational Processes and the Facilitating

Environment. International Universities Press.

Yalom, I. (1980) Existential Psychotherapy. Basic Books.

Sylvia Flescher

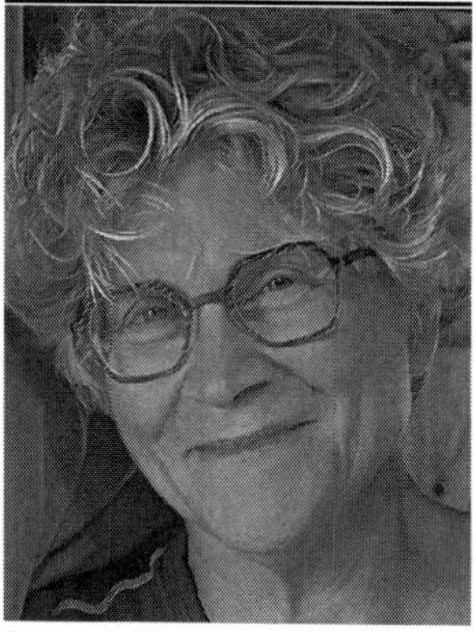

SYLVIA FLESCHER, M.D. calls herself a "survivor of the New York Psychoanalytic Institute." On faculty at Mount Sinai Medical Center in NYC, she is past-President of the New Jersey Psychoanalytic Society. She is now moving towards retirement after nearly half a century in the field. She lives with her husband and three cats in Bergen County, N.J. and is currently enjoying her new role as grandmother to her two-year old grandson, Jake.

This is a chapter from Dr. Flescher's forthcoming memoir, entitled *The Reluctant Psychoanalyst: a Daughter's Memoir,* to be published in August 2026 by SheWritesPress and distributed by Simon and Schuster.

Of Pens and Swords

I'M AT LUNCH WITH A FELLOW PSYCHOANALYST, AND THE FAMILIAR SONG OF SELF-DOUBT IS PLAYING IN MY HEAD: *He's the real deal and I'm just a sham. He can talk the psychoanalytic talk with such assurance, while I trail off into generalities to cover up my poor memory and lousy grasp of theory. He's an academic, with published papers to his name, teaching courses with scholarly bibliographies. His office is lined floor-to-ceiling with books, all of which he has surely read and can confidently quote from. It's only a matter of time before I'm found out.*

I share with him a troubling event that occurred in my office the preceding week. I feel obliged to confess what happened, possibly to write about my grave technical gaffe, thereby proving to the world how incompetent I am. In my head, I continue to catastrophize: my practice will dwindle to nothing, and I'll be reduced to writing prescriptions at a clinic. Soon enough, I'll be broke and homeless.

I briefly sketch out the clinical situation. My patient, Mr. B., in the third year of a four-times-a-week analysis, perpetually berates himself for not being a good father or a good husband. We're meeting on Monday, after my one-week vacation. In the run-up to the trip, I have misplaced my mailbox key: an example of a "parapraxis." Often as I prepare for a trip, my separation anxiety disorganizes me and I'm likely to lose or forget something. Without my key, I can't open my mailbox. As my patient is deep into the telling of an erotically charged dream, I hear the mailman enter the lobby and begin to distribute the mail into our mailboxes. I say, "Excuse me," stand up and exit the room into the lobby to ask for my mail, explaining about the lost key. A moment later, I

> "What kind of analyst would do a thing like that?" My friend smiles and says in a warm, teasing tone, "I think you should fall on your sword."

return, a week's mail clutched in my arms. Why does this seem so important to me? Partly because I'm waiting for several substantial checks from patients to replenish my dwindling bank account.

Mr. B. becomes furious that I interrupted the session, leaving him so abruptly. I try hard not to feel defensive, and to remain open to exploring Mr. B.'s reaction.

Later I realize that this could have been an unconscious repetition of a moment in my own analysis, when Dr. N. suddenly got up without a word, and left. I felt puzzled at first, then abandoned and frightened. When she returned a few moments later and I described what I'd experienced, she said in a tone I heard as irritated, "Didn't you hear the doorbell?" I had not.

The 30-second interaction with my patient carries in it so many potential avenues to be mined that I feel inclined to try to write about it; but I ask my colleague, literally covering my eyes in shame, "What kind of analyst would do a thing like that?" My friend smiles and says in a warm, teasing tone, "I think you should fall on your sword."

I laugh with him and at myself, letting the playful words sink in. They've taken me totally by surprise. Not only is he not judging me, he's humorously and artfully reminding me that I needn't take myself so seriously. For days afterward, his words repeat in my mind. I feel my shoulders drop away from their habitual position close to my ears. And in the space that he's created for me there is now room to hold onto a more tolerant and forgiving view of myself and my analytic abilities. He has effectively detoxified my feeling of shame, allowing me instead to stay in a stance of neutral—or better yet, benevolent—curiosity. If I collapse the space for analytic exploration with a flurry of self-recrimination, I can't remain curious about what this disruption might mean for me and for my patient.

My friend's gentle teasing makes me aware of my excessive expectations and undue anxiety. After all, this was not a life-and-death error. I'm not a Samurai warrior who has brought unspeakable dishonor onto myself, my family, my nation, my emperor! If I write about this clinical moment, maybe I won't be committing professional *hara-kiri*, but joining instead with other clinician-writers who candidly and courageously expose their humanity and fallibility. Perhaps this interaction—running out on my patient and then not getting overly defensive, indeed tolerating his anger, without withdrawing or retaliating—will provide us with a new way of relating. By modeling for my patient that I'm fallible, that I can acknowledge my error, accept his angry disappointment in me and move past it, maybe I can help him be more forgiving of himself.

Neither he nor I have to be perfect.

Matthew Varley

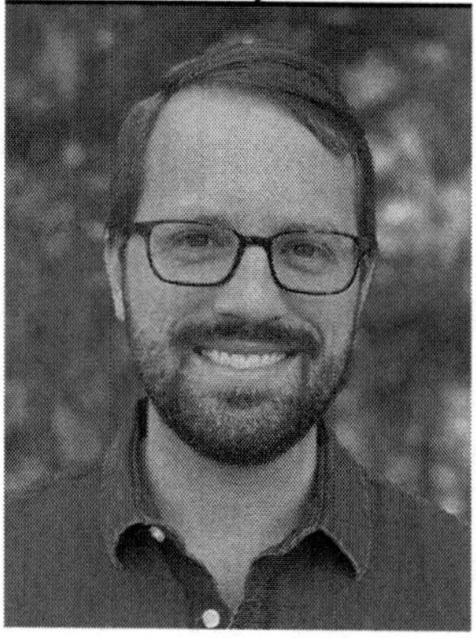

MATTHEW VARLEY, PHD works with adolescents, adults, couples and families in private practice in Durham, NC. He has special interests in myths and archetypes, men's development, and psychedelic-assisted therapy. This is his first contribution to *Voices*. *msvarley@gmail.com*

Selling Bliss

IT WAS AN UNUSUAL CRAIGSLIST JOB POSTING FOR MY SOUTHERN HOMETOWN: "ORGANIC FOOD MANUFACTURER SEEKS SALES REPRESENTATIVE." Sales seemed intimidating to me, an introvert who had imagined a career teaching or writing. But I was intrigued by the company called Pure Bliss, I like to eat, and I was beginning to feel desperate. Instead of drafting yet another cover letter, I decided to call. The owner, Jon, answered. I told him I was a recent college graduate and admitted my major, religious studies, which I had come to view as a liability in my job search. "Oh," Jon replied, "I'm a Hare Krishna devotee." He invited me in for an interview.

I put on a suit and tried to imagine myself a salesperson. I left for the interview in ample time but hit a road closure and arrived twenty minutes late, stressed, apologetic and assuming it was over. But Jon and his business partner, Antonio, were surprisingly sympathetic. The company occupied a suite in a nondescript office park with no sign on the door. There were three plain offices and a hallway tripling as a kitchen, breakroom and storage space. A door at the end of the hall opened to a warehouse converted into a commercial kitchen. Baking spice aromas wafted from giant ovens. Cooling racks parked alongside pallets of oats, nuts, sweeteners and dried fruit. I met a few workers mixing granola in bath-size plastic tubs.

Then I sat with Jon and Antonio in a windowless office for an interview. I don't recall how I answered the stock question: "Tell us about your weaknesses." But an honest response would have been something like: "I have no idea what I'm doing with my life or why I'm in-

"We shook hands. I wasn't at all confident I would get the job, and not sure at all I wanted it, but a few days later Jon made me an offer.."

terviewing for a job selling granola." I tried to bend my experience to appear suitable for sales, leaning, for example, on cold-calling leads as a campus newspaper reporter (my least favorite part). We shook hands. I wasn't at all confident I would get the job, and not sure at all I wanted it, but a few days later Jon made me an offer. I accepted with a mix of emotions: gratitude for the opportunity, relief the job search was over, shock I would be doing this particular job, and deep uncertainty about my first shaky step into adulthood.

I had graduated from a prestigious university in the spring, full of oblivious confidence in my potential and the many good opportunities I imagined awaiting me. The global financial crisis registered only as a headline my senior year, while I busied myself with writing an honors thesis, partying, and relishing the rhythms of college life. For most of my 23 years, I had been told and believed I was special. Everything about my academic life reinforced this, and I did little to prepare to enter a world I imagined wide open for my arrival. Maybe I would write for a major publication, work for a name-brand nonprofit, or teach in a private school while deciding if I wanted to go to graduate school in the humanities or study law. I had solid credentials, lots of interests, and naïve optimism about the future.

Then I took a hard fall out of the ivory tower, passing the summer of 2009 in my childhood bedroom, writing cover letters and arranging "networking meetings" with loose connections. These felt forced and went nowhere. Rejections from Teach for America and private schools, PBS and small-town newspapers, and charities large and small arrived in my inbox. Or, more often, I received no response. Clearly, I wasn't interested in business—I wanted to do something creative, intellectually challenging, or good in the world according to me. But as summer cooled into fall, my goal shifted to moving out of my parents' house, and I turned to local jobs posted on Craigslist. When I told my parents I had taken the granola job, my mom was typically encouraging. My father looked down, avoiding my eyes. I appreciated his effort to hold back criticism, but he didn't have to say anything.

Jon gave me the front office, the one with a window, which doubled as a storage room packed floor-to-ceiling with packaged granola, energy bars, and snack mixes. On my first day, I assembled a big-box desk and chair, then began the first of several shifts working production in the warehouse. I learned not just how the products were made, but the spirit in which the company made them. As a Hare Krishna devotee, Jon made prasadam – food as a religious sacrament. Before a batch of anything was tasted or packaged, Jon placed a few morsels on a bookshelf altar in his office. He rang a bell, bowed in prayer, and offered the food to Krishna. Like the communion ritual, this sacralized the food and assured spiritual benefits to anyone who consumed it. And this philosophy made the company's work a devotional practice whose chief goals were non-material. We didn't advertise our products as blessed, but it made a difference in how they were made and showed me an example of how a business could be led by purpose.

I had a computer, a phone, and a list of natural food retailers across the USA. Jon handled existing accounts; it was my job to cold-call potential new customers, send product samples, and follow up to make sales. I had a small base salary plus a small commission. The work was nerve-wracking at first; the anxiety abated over time, but it never disappeared. "Hello, this is Matt from Pure Bliss," I would say. "May I please speak to the buyer? Are you open to bringing in new products? Can I send you samples of our best-sellers?" I could never anticipate who would answer the phone or what kind of reception I would get. The responses ran a full gamut from warm to hostile, expansive to brusque, grateful to condescending. But I did believe in the products surrounding me in the cramped storage-office. They were truly delicious: granolas made with fresh bananas and cinnamon, peanut butter and chocolate; hearty and chewy snack bars made with oats, dates and coconut; sweet and spicy nut mixes. All of it was made with simple and organic ingredients, by hand, right down the hallway. I could smell it baking while I dialed.

"The work was nerve-wracking at first; the anxiety abated over time, but it never disappeared."

Still, I had to muster courage to make the initial calls - bothering people at work! - and even more to call back a week later and try to close. "Can I go ahead and send you two cases of our top-selling granolas and a case each of our energy bars"? It went against my nature to be so direct but surprisingly often, the answer was "yes." Jon had coached me on a quirk of human psychology: people often don't know what they want (I could relate!); we can sometimes help them by removing decisions and simply telling them. Of course I was often rejected. I was an amateur salesperson for an unknown brand among a vast field of competitors. But here too, Jon offered wisdom. "We show up, do our job the best we can, and don't get too attached to the outcome," he counseled, drawing on the wisdom of the Bhagavad Gita. "That part is ultimately not under our control."

Jon was not the mentor I could have, or would have, sought out. Though he came from considerably less privilege than me, he could perhaps relate to my lost-soul stage, which he too experienced in youth until reading the Gita on the Appalachian Trail. Instead of college, he moved into an ashram to cook, pray, and live in community for a decade. When he left, his guru told him it was better to be self-employed than work for someone else, so he applied his culinary skills and started the company with a friend and a credit card. He had no formal business training and was undercapitalized in a competitive, low-margin market. He was figuring it out as he went along - and making it - though the path was paved with trial-and-error. I knew considerably less than he did but nevertheless felt free to criticize things I saw lacking at the company. No doubt much of this was a projection of my own discomfort with my station, and a dream the business could suddenly make it (and me) big. The attachment to outcome wasn't easy to release.

When I criticized a sloppy record-keeping system leading to missed orders, and an incoherent marketing strategy limiting our visibility, Jon listened openly to my feedback. He made me feel seen and appreciated, and he made changes. We collaborated to design new packages, write marketing copy, start social media campaigns, and modify the flavors and names of several new products. These parts of the job I truly enjoyed, and I began to take pride in our scrappy, gourmet, underdog business. Also, I made

"Many young graduates are encouraged to 'seek out mentors.' My experience taught me to be open to mentors I might not imagine or recognize at first."

enough money to move out of my parent's house. Still, the long afternoons of cold calling were tedious. While I pounded coffee, Jon, who forswore all intoxicants, often napped face-down on his desk. He hired and fired three other salespeople during my 2.5-year tenure. Once, Jon used the company kitchen to prepare a huge batch of yogurt for a religious festival. It sat culturing for a week in a twenty-gallon plastic tub. The day of the fest, I watched him roll it past my office on a cart and over the front door threshold, then heard a crash. I walked outside in time to see the white tidal wave ooze across the parking lot. Jon shouted his usual frustrated exclamation: "Krishna!" But he was quick to chalk up the mishap up to his usual clumsiness. I thought about how angry I would have been at myself in his position, and I admired his self-deprecating grace.

Meanwhile, in my free time, I kept trying to discern what might be next. One afternoon on my lunch break, I paced the parking lot talking to my old college advisor, wondering if I had made a mistake not to pursue graduate school in religious studies, and was it too late? I took the LSAT, was accepted to law school, and decided not to enroll because it still didn't feel like my path. I applied for another sales job, at a company everyone knows in California, flew out for an interview, and was rejected. I started tutoring in the evenings, first for a family friend and then for a local agency. And I expanded the scope of my networking meetings to include a neighbor, Elaine, who was a therapist. She talked about her job in ways that truly appealed to me, and she gently suggested I might benefit from therapy myself. Once I got started with her referral, Don, things started to change. I decided to pursue tutoring full time and eventually graduate school in counseling. On my last day, Jon made homemade pizza (even better than his granola) which everyone gathered in the hallway-breakroom to enjoy. Then he sent me off well-nourished for my journey.

If I had known sooner where I was going after college, I would have avoided substantial stress, and I might be further along in my career as a psychologist today. Instead, I was humbled and opened to experiences and people I would never have otherwise encountered, and who continue to loom large in my psyche. Many young graduates are encouraged to "seek out mentors." My experience taught me to be open to mentors I might not imagine or recognize at first. Jon saw potential in me when I was struggling. He gave me a chance to learn and grow into a role I never imagined for myself, taught me how to be more direct with people, and gave me many daily opportunities to practice assertiveness. He modeled a way of being serious about work without taking himself too seriously, and he possessed a sense of devotion and spiritual meaning in life to which I continue to aspire. I still don't think I would laugh at myself if I spilled all that yogurt.

Commentary

I read "Selling Bliss" as a short story of discovery and self discovery, written in retrospect. However, the story of how the author was gently mentored into his decision to become a psychotherapist is constructed so that it unfolds as he experienced it, slowly, accumulatively and without knowing the outcome.

As such, if read too literally, we may remain clueless until the very end as to how his journey relates to becoming a psychotherapist, rather than, say, a salesperson, or owner of a small company selling products that reflect his values. (Both outcomes are somewhat confusingly reflected in the title which would be an odd way indeed to refer to the practice of psychotherapy.) The often exquisite and loving attention to physical details of person, place and daily life, promote a sense of universality, of a mentoring process that could apply to any career decision. The result can be disorienting given the context of a clinical journal: this article would be at equally at home in a collection of short stories on the power of mentoring.

Another way of putting this is to say that the article requires the reader to do some work to realize that that each lesson learned makes the author not only better at selling "Bliss" but also a good candidate for the experience and practice of psychotherapy and probably a better person. For example, Jon addresses his fears of getting rejected when making cold calls by advising that "we show up, do our job the best we can, and don't get too attached to the outcome." Fine advice for salespeople, psychotherapists and life. Or, as Adam Phillips puts it, "The psychoanalyst... must ask herself not, Am I being a good analyst... have I said the right thing? But, What kind of person do I want to be?"

—Rhona Engels *rhonae1@gmail.com*

Commentary

This author had me at "I have no idea what I'm doing with my life or why I'm interviewing for a job selling granola." Actually, he had me at "religious studies." I have a soft spot in my heart for anyone whose college major rendered them unemployable upon graduation. I figured I could always live in my car if a B.A. in Philosophy didn't get me any traction on the job market. But that was in 1993. Committing to something that speaks deeply to the mind and spirit in 2009 seems that much more reckless. Bravo!

Bravo as well for being open to unexpected experiences and letting them matter. Matt's boss, Jon, offers a classic piece of wisdom: "We show up, do our job the best we can, and don't get too attached to the outcome." Jon really walks the walk. This is not just Non-attachment; this is a massive amount of yogurt sliding onto parking lot pavement. Gross.

Jon also offers a different portrait of adulthood than Matt had at home. When I was his age, ideas about Life became valid once I could triangulate them: my therapist, my yoga teacher, and my boss couldn't all be wrong. And some of that wisdom makes its way into my work to this day. I don't know him (hi, Matt!), but I know I'd like to. I love an introvert, I love a thoughtful person who can write well, and I love a person with respect for the unlikely moments on their journey.

—Stephanie Spalding

Morning Paper (November 6, 2024)

Tom Large
tomlarge14@gmail.com

Outside for the morning paper,
a somber stillness everywhere,
makes me wonder, has Baltimore been evacuated?
A single bird calls from the park across the street,
one hesitant squawk
that goes unanswered.
I listen to it echo in the quiet of the morning.
To my nearly blind eyes
The eastern sky, smudges of pale blue and orange,
looks like Dundalk is burning.
I've come for the paper but that's only an excuse
to be in the open and feel the first stirrings of a breeze,
cool and fresh in the empty street.
This peace, broken by the day's first stirrings,
deserves my witness, as the curtain goes up
on a future I'm not prepared for.
The newspaper on the grass comes wrapped in plastic
so the print isn't spoiled by the morning dew.
For his thoughtfulness I'm grateful to the delivery man,
though today I won't read even the headlines.
There are more bird calls now,
some answering one another
some laying down their solo melodies.
When the last newspapers cease to print
because honest journalists are in prison
and the only glow on the horizon
comes from mounds of books burning,
I will keep going outside before sun up,
to take heart from those few birds
brave enough to sing out in the dark.

Speechless

Tom Large

I have nothing to say today,
not one word about the latest mass shooting
or the atrocities in Ukraine.
I have nothing to say about climate change
or the recent virus surge,
not one word.
If my neighbor, Dave, invites me yet again
into a political conversation,
I will say, "Sorry, Dave, I'm late for a meeting,"
and hurriedly walk away.
If a colleague at the office says,
"Finally they've convicted him of something,"
I will say, "I'm all for politicians with convictions."
If the clerk at my local library
says, "Did you hear Mark Twain is banned in Birmingham?"
I will only nod and hurry home.
Sitting by this open window
on this fine summer morning,
I'll let the sparrows in the linden trees,
that are chirping with real enthusiasm,
do all the talking.

Marilyn Schwartz

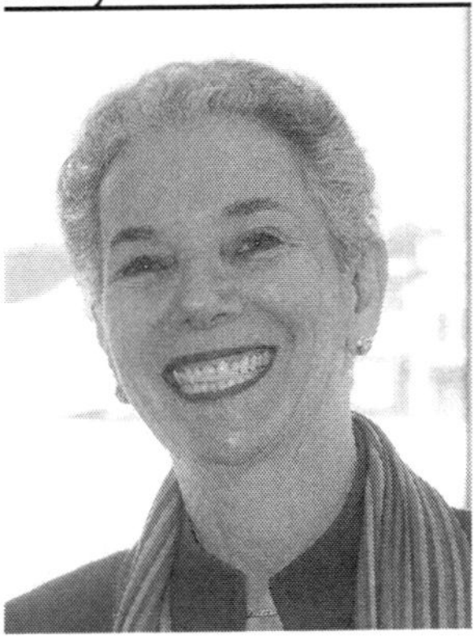

Marilyn Schwartz, PhD, has been a psychologist in private practice for 50 years in DC. She co-directed the Adult ADHD Center of Washington and has been a psychologist consultant to the Smithsonian Institution. She loves wrestling with ethical dilemmas, being former chair of the AAP Ethics Committee from 2011 to 2022 and presenting 23 different ethics workshops at AAP meetings.
drmarilynschwartz@gmail.com

Developing the Person of the Therapist—
A Tradition Taught Through the Stories We Tell

As I've contemplated the importance of seasoned therapists passing down their traditions, knowledge, and wisdom to the next generations of therapists, I'm reminded of the Jewish expression "l'dor v'dor" (from generation to generation). This concept from the Torah emphasizes one's responsibility to transmit knowledge, beliefs, customs, and stories to future generations, highlighting the importance of intergenerational connections and support.

This reminds me of my role as a parent and grandparent, sharing stories that convey traditions and values that are held by my family and myself personally. These stories are carefully tailored to each child's age, often relating experiences from when I was their age. In my view, it is not only important to locate myself in the story, but especially to share how I may have learned an important lesson from a mistake I've made. Owning one's struggles in a story allows an identification and sharing of wisdom between generations, whether the audience is your children, grandchildren, or younger colleagues.

As an example, when my children and grandchildren entered adolescence, I loved telling the story about my struggle with resisting peer pressure. At sixteen, as a counselor in training at summer camp, I couldn't resist following the lead of older counselors, sneaking out of camp through the woods to the nearby town, Thurmont, MD. Wanting to be cool, I went along with purchasing alcohol illegally and getting horribly drunk for the first time in my life. On our return, we got lost in the woods, and next thing we knew, we were surrounded by soldiers pointing automatic weapons at us, having inadvertently found our way onto the grounds of Camp David, the presidential retreat. Learning that your mother or grandmother got arrested at sixteen communicates a powerful cautionary tale about exercising good judgment and resisting peer pressure.

Storytelling may be one of the most effective ways to convey my belief in the centrality of the therapist as a critical factor in the psychotherapeutic relationship and its effectiveness. This belief and the related tradition of developing the person of the therapist have been core values of my professional organization, the American Academy of Psychotherapists (AAP). Reflecting on my 45+ years membership in this organization and now being an elder, I can recognize the importance of stories shared by more seasoned members in my early career and those I've repeatedly told younger colleagues, passing down this belief in the centrality of the therapist and the tradition of developing the person of the therapist. Here are examples of five different kinds of stories:

A Story About You

Perhaps the most important story told by mentors and professional elders is about you—a story you may not quite know, but hearing it may make all the difference in how you develop as a therapist. One such story was told to me by an early supervisor and mentor, Dr. Sheldon Kopp. Shelly, as he was known to a generation of therapists he supervised in the 70s, and 80s, was regarded as a therapist guru for his prolific writing about psychotherapy and his unique manner of group supervision. If you were his supervisee and wanted a consultation around a client, Shelly required you to bring your client to the group session so that he could observe you interacting with your client in real time. Unlike other supervisors, Shelly focused on your way of being present in the relationship rather than primarily on the client's dynamics or pathology.

After observing my work with clients, Shelly repeatedly told me, "Marilyn, stop going into your head, trust your intuition. You're always on your mark when you do so." He explained that I should trust my intuition because it held, not only my knowledge and empathy, but, more importantly, the unique trait he saw in me - how my whirling dervish mind could generate creative ideas to reframe the client's issues and provide insight. His story about me built my confidence in my clinical judgment and helped me develop my unique therapeutic style.

As the Talmud saying goes, "behind every blade of grass, there is an angel that says: grow, grow". Perhaps, the greatest gift we can give to younger therapists is a story about themselves: what aspect of their unique personhood can be nurtured and developed so they can become their most effective therapeutic self.

The Lessons Our Clients Teach Us

Lessons from our clients can, also, become powerful stories about the centrality and development of the therapist. Here's an example of how a client taught me an invaluable lesson about self-care and its importance in supporting clients through their most challenging therapeutic moments.

After several years of therapy, a client finally felt safe enough to address her childhood history of physical and sexual abuse. She arrived at this pivotal session with the largest bouquet I'd ever seen, explaining it was to "protect me from the horror" of hear-

As the Talmudic saying goes, "behind every blade of grass there is an angel that says: Grow. Grow." Perhaps the greatest gift we can give to younger therapists is a story about themselves.

ing about her traumatic experiences. In subsequent sessions, we would both take breaks to look at these magnificent bouquets she brought, helping us to remain grounded. As Freud warned, "the analyst must deal with hazardous materials that require special precautions, lest the handler be gravely injured" (Freud, 1937/1964, p. 249).

I remain deeply grateful for this lesson in self-care and have shared it with many. Because of our centrality in the therapeutic relationship, we must attend to our self-care to remain fully present and effective. Also, in processing and showing gratitude to the client for her "gift" of the bouquets, I came to understand the value of mutual caretaking in the therapeutic relationship, especially at times when undertaking deeper work.

Our Biggest Regret Story

Another impactful narrative is our "biggest regret" as a therapist. I imagine every therapist must have one. Mine involves a long-term client, a 40-year-old husband and father of two young children, who was suddenly hospitalized with a brain bleed several hours from our city and subsequently died. I deeply regret not reaching out to him to see if he would have wanted me to visit him in the hospital. I imagine he wouldn't have felt comfortable asking me to make the long trip to see him, but it was certainly a trip I would have made given the nature of our long and loving relationship.

In hindsight, I regret being too hesitant to act on my deep feelings of caring for this client, which I believe were mutual. Did I fail to recognize the importance to him of our relationship? When sharing this story, I always add that I wish I had followed the advice attributed to Dr. Karl Menninger: "When in doubt, be human."

Our Story About an Ethical Misstep

Confessional stories about struggling with an ethical dilemma uniquely convey the importance of the therapist's development in the ethical realm. Beyond being present, our trustworthiness, honesty, reliability, and ethical conduct create the safe harbor necessary for therapeutic work. Sharing a story about wrestling with an ethical dilemma or even a significant mistake offers valuable lessons about the personal and professional growth required when we hold this position of centrality in the therapeutic relationship.

My confession: Early in my career, I seriously breached a client's confidentiality. The client mentioned that one of my colleagues was likely having an affair and separating from their spouse. Noting my surprise, the client added, "Everyone knows about this." Weeks later, during dinner with another colleague after an exhausting workday, I thoughtlessly remarked, "Can you believe Dr. X is separating from his wife?" This colleague, a close friend of Dr. X, looked surprised and asked, "How do you know? No one knows about this."

Apparently, the client had misspoken, and I was caught in a terrible ethical dilemma of how to explain how I knew about this. Fortunately, this breach of confidentiality had no serious consequences, as I was fortunate that it occurred with a trusted colleague, with whom I was able to process my actions, feelings, and learnings from this breach. But the experience taught me the invaluable lesson about the absolute duty of maintaining confidentiality and upholding other ethical requirements that accompany our central role in the therapeutic relationship.

Appropriating Stories and Best Lines

Another rich source of storytelling for passing down our core beliefs and traditions about psychotherapy comes from the stories and best lines we appropriate from others. For decades, I've kept a small collection of these in the side pocket of my briefcase—quotes, anecdotes, and sayings that have inspired me and that I often share with both clients and colleagues.

One of my favorite stories is The Starfish Story (Eiseley, 1969), which I first heard from a psychiatrist and longtime AAP member, the late Dr. Stephen Howard. It's about an old man walking along the beach, tossing stranded starfish, among hundreds of them, back into the sea one at a time. When a passerby questions why he bothers, saying that there are so many on the beach that it won't make any difference no matter how many he throws back in the sea, the old man replies, "It makes a difference to that one."

I've returned to this story, or shared it with others, time and again—especially during those moments when the work feels overwhelming or when it seems futile that we're helping only one person at a time. This story serves as a powerful reminder that what we do matters deeply to that one client—and at times, it may even be lifesaving.

Even simple lines, passed down through colleagues, can hold extraordinary meaning. Just recently, I heard someone quote this same colleague, Dr. Stephen Howard, as saying: "Although you may feel frustrated or bored with a client who seems not to be making progress, it may be that your presence—your listening and your caring—is what's saving their life."

Bidirectional Storytelling

I hope my examples convey the value of storytelling in transmitting to younger generations of therapists' hard-won beliefs and traditions, like the centrality of the therapist, and developing the person of the therapist. However, I also recognize that this cross-generational conversation can work both ways—seasoned therapists can learn substantially from stories told by younger colleagues.

Early and mid-career therapists bring fresh perspectives shaped by emerging trends and new approaches. For instance, newer therapists might draw more readily on neuroscience research, using concepts like neuroplasticity and trauma's impact on the nervous system to inform interventions. In addition, as training today places a strong emphasis on cultural humility, intersectionality, and social justice, newer therapists may have a more intentional focus on understanding how identity, privilege, and oppression affect mental health and the therapeutic relationship.

As an example of this, I greatly appreciated when a newly licensed therapist in a workshop I presented at a recent meeting shared with me and the predominantly seasoned therapists in the room the story of their struggle dealing with professional presentations like mine in which the material and research that supports it are based on categorizing therapists in terms of the binary of male and female. As they explained, unless this bias is acknowledged and addressed in research, this approach promotes heteronormativity, i.e., the view that heterosexuality is the norm or preferred sexual orientation. Also, as an important part of the story, they bravely shared this causes therapists like themselves, who are not gender identified as male or female, to feel less accepted in professional spaces. If we remain open and take the time to listen, therapists of every generation have valuable stories and lessons to share that can foster our development and help us become our best therapist selves.

References:

Eiseley, L. (1969). The star thrower. In The unexpected universe (pp. 65–76). Harcourt Brace Jovanovich.

Freud, S. (1964). Analysis terminable and interminable (J. Strachey, Trans.). In J. Strachey (Ed.), The standard edition of the complete psychological works of Sigmund Freud (Vol. 23, p. 249). Hogarth Press. (Original work published 1937)

Menninger, K. (n.d.). Quote attributed to Karl Menninger. Source of original work not verifiable.

"If you look deeply into the palm of your hand, you will see your parents and all generations of your ancestors. All of them are alive in this moment. Each is present in your body. You are the continuation of each of these people." —Thich Nhat Hanh

Edward H. Jacobs

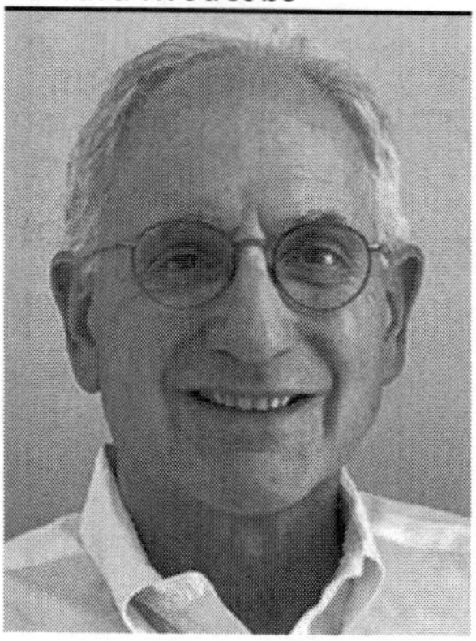

Edward H. Jacobs, PhD, is a New England-based psychologist and writer. His novel, *Splintered River*—a literary political drama—was published this fall. His literary work (short stories, poetry, memoir) has appeared in several journals. He has published two books on parenting children with ADHD, peer-reviewed papers on self psychology, family therapy, chronic pain, learning disabilities and neurofeedback, and articles for the general public on psychological topics, and he has been a contributing book review editor for the *American Journal of Psychotherapy*. He has served on the clinical faculty of Harvard Medical School. His work can be seen at *www.ehjacobsauthor.com*.

A Psychologist Looks Back

When I began my graduate training some forty-seven years ago, I knew, somewhere in the back of my mind, that there would come a final day of work, where my mind would not center on the problem right before me, but on the entire expanse of my professional enterprise. But, like so many things we take on in our youth, that day seemed far off, to be dealt with "when the time came."

And, since I had worked in mental health for several years prior to my graduate training, I knew, going into the field, that any meaningful measure of success, for me, would not be quantifiable and verifiable in the ways it might be for my peers who went into business, or sales, or even law: how much money made (for self or for clients), how many cases won or lost, how many units sold, how many awards earned or platitudes achieved (for how many consecutive years did one make "Winners' Circle," or "President's Circle" or "Platinum Level"?). I was in a private practice that I had established and built over the thirty-seven years, for which I did not keep statistics. Although, even if I had, outcome measures in mental health are notoriously unreliable and based on the word of the clinician and/or the patient, dependent on subjectivity, mostly short-term in nature and, by necessity, concrete and specific in ways that can overlook the intangibles of clinical work. Although there were patients whose progress could be quantified, there were many whose progress defied quantification. I spent many hours, in both community mental health and in private practice, filling out forms that documented "progress" in order to get continuing services approved for patients

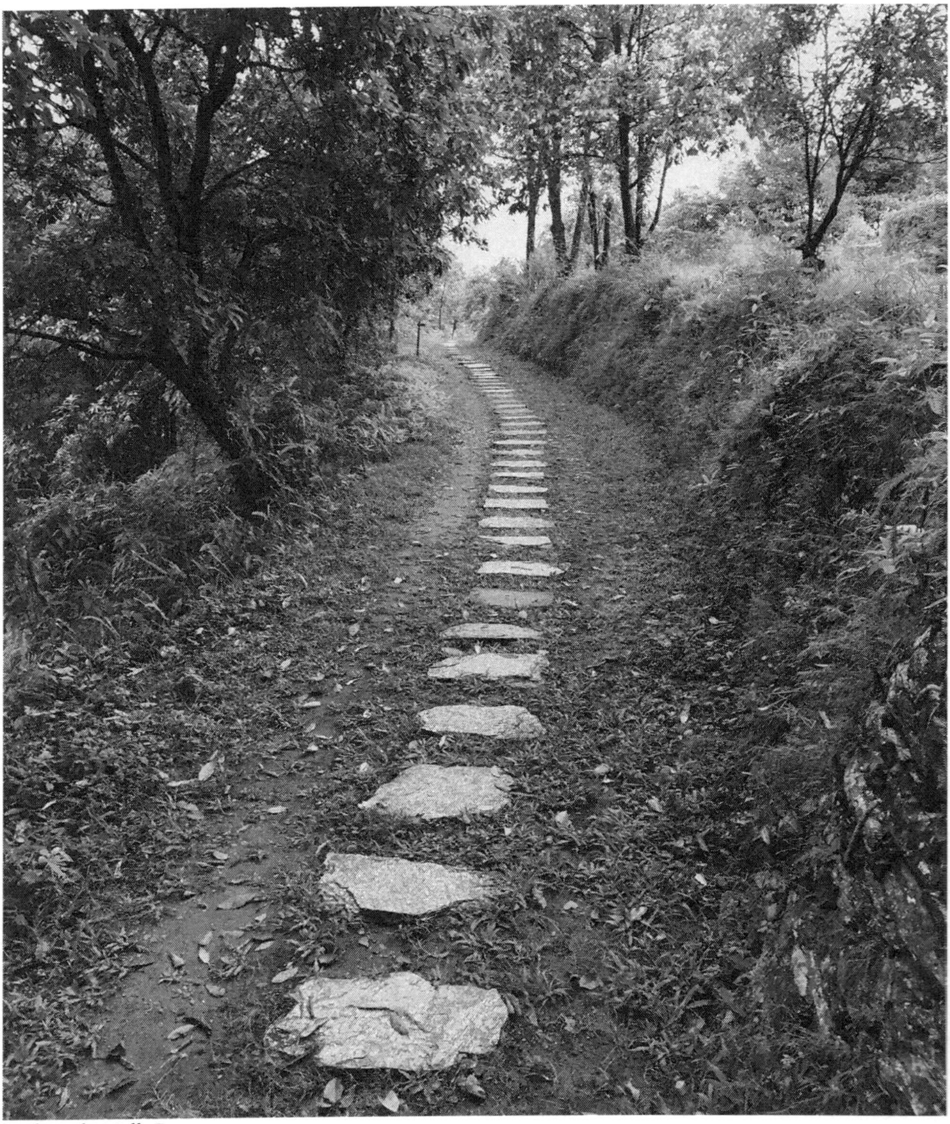

Pathway by Molly Donovan

who badly needed them, people I was afraid would fall apart or suffer if denied treatment, and for whom I could not articulate in any specific, concrete and time-defined way the good our work had done (except that, perhaps, they had not gotten worse, committed suicide, beaten their child or gotten themselves arrested). I just knew that they had been helped and that they needed continued services. How was I so sure, you might ask? Maybe they weren't progressing, maybe they would have done just as well without me or done better with another therapist. And you would be correct in posing those questions. Maybe their affect seemed improved some small percentage of the time. Maybe they spoke with some small degree of insight into their behavior, maybe they just kept a greater percentage of their appointments than they had the year before.

I did not have scales to precisely measure these factors and do comparisons demonstrating whether these improvements were statistically significant.

And, as far as technique, the pioneering psychologist Carl Rogers found that successful psychotherapy depends on the qualities of warmth, genuineness and empathy in the therapist, and that this was both true and necessary no matter the specific techniques employed or the theoretical orientation subscribed to by the therapist. So, although I could cite specific things I might have done that were therapeutic, was it really just my therapeutic presence and manner that counted after all? We sit in a room with a patient or patients, with the door closed and no one observing. How can we possibly assess our work objectively? And yet, change, we believe, happens.

In the self-appraisal of my work this is what I know. I made a living, I trained at reputable institutions, I worked in a variety of settings, I established and maintained a successful practice, I employed, supervised, mentored and trained other clinicians, I published in the field, I taught and lectured, I had a constant stream of referrals from other professionals and from the public at large, and I had thousands of patients walk through my doors, some belonging to families spanning multiple generations of self-referral. One would think that I would feel justified in thinking: Job well done! Time to move on. But I'm a psychologist and, by both temperament and training, I simply cannot do that.

The important over-arching question for me is: did I help people? I remember one of my graduate school professors saying that he was surprised that not one of the prospective students he interviewed for admission asked him how many people he had cured, although I ponder if, in this business, there really is such a thing as "cure." The psychiatrist Thomas Szasz insisted that there is no such thing as "mental illness," that what we are looking at are "problems in living." So, perhaps a better notion than "cure" would be: were my patients' lives better as a result of working with me? I think I can answer this unequivocally in the affirmative, based on my years of training, experience, supervision, and feedback from patients and colleagues. I remember being plagued by self-doubt during my clinical internship, and one of my supervisors—a woman not given to artifice or hyperbole—telling me that my relationship with my patients was therapeutic and that they knew it. I remember very little of what else was said to me during that year, but that has stuck.

Yet, I am still haunted by memories of people I could not help: the adolescents I lost patience with, the patients who knew how to press my buttons and engender internal anxiety, anger or self-doubt, people with personalities or ways of being in the world that set off irrational reactions from deep within me about which I had limited understanding or control, the couples with whom I had difficulty being neutral and objective, the patients I just wanted to "shake" but wasn't sure how to confront.

I keep hearing how important self-care is to help a therapist maintain emotional balance and objectivity. It turns out that rest, sleep, vacation and fun do not always come about at the right time. I remember so many mornings feeling overwhelmed, waking up and looking at the day, at the number of patients I had scheduled, at the reports I had to get out and the phone calls I had to return, at the insurance companies and former patients I had to chase for payment, at the paperwork I had to do, at the sheer number of hours that I had to be "on" while being scrutinized by patients as I tried to understand them—dealing with their anger and tension around needs I could not meet (made un-

"The important, overarching question for me is:

Did I help people?

necessarily more difficult with my life-long concern with being liked), and having to force myself to stay alert and even awake at times when I was tired, overwhelmed or distracted. There were times when I just didn't want to be there, being preoccupied with some personal or family matter or obsessing about some technical or computer problem that was driving me crazy and I just wanted to fix. There were times that I was hungry and could only think of the meal I wanted to eat when I was done being a therapist for the day. For all these lapses, as human as they are, I still feel guilty.

But, even if I give myself credit for helping many people lead better lives, I still have the question of whether I helped them enough. I consulted with many clinicians over the course of my career, whom I admired for their insight, compassion or patience, or simply for their ability to be present for their patients, and I wished that I could emulate those characteristics myself. Could I have been mindful enough to have embodied these qualities more consistently? Could I have acquired these qualities through additional training? I have never answered these questions to my satisfaction. My question relates to the issue of whether great therapists are born or made. I believe that people are who they are and, no matter what changes they make in their lives, their basic personality remains. So, can a therapist with a certain temperament really grow beyond the limitations of that temperament? Can one use training and experience to make oneself more empathic, more connected, more patient, more insightful? I believe that they can, but to what extent? At what point, to paraphrase D.W. Winnicott, is one a "good enough" therapist? Are there people who are just not capable of getting there (and might I be one of them)?

Another question arises for me: do the traits we develop as therapists transfer to our personal lives? I remember telling a family member of mine who accused me of being impatient that I had to be patient in order to do the work that I did. So, why was it difficult to incorporate this quality into my family self?

Apropos of the above, did I have enough insight to get out of my own way when I had to? I know I did so with regard to couples therapy. Couples therapy had interested me because it seemed to combine the best of psychodynamic and systems work. However, I found myself overwhelmed by the "he said/she said" dynamics and felt like a referee who was being pulled in different directions by sides that were not interested in listening so much as they were interested in being listened to. I remember one couple whom I failed to help and with whom I felt particularly helpless. They recontacted me after termination, asking to work with me again, claiming that they had agreed on a place to begin and from which to build. I initially declined. After some persuasion on their part, I agreed to re-engage, and had an even more frustrating and disappointing experience. Unbeknownst to me, the stakes in their marriage had intensified. Although their new starting point for therapy was rather concrete—agreeing on a budget—the husband had for the most part moved out and was working in another city during the week and he had developed a relationship with a female colleague to whom he had introduced his daughter, without the mother's permission. So, the stakes had risen even higher, and focusing on their "starting point" was like discussing the color of the dining room in a house that, once beset by storm, was now in the midst of a tornado.

I realized that my working with couples re-enacted my childhood experience of feeling helpless, caught between two parents who were perpetually feuding, and that no amount of training, supervision, insight and experience was going to "cure" me of this. Eventually, I became wise enough to refer all the couples that came my way to my wife, who loves working with couples, and who is much more emotionally balanced than I am.

I also continually struggled with whether I was doing therapy the "right" way. The field of psychology is replete with so many, at times overlapping, at times contradictory, schools of thought, each with its own model for understanding human behavior and its own techniques for addressing human problems and suffering. One must choose or not choose. Not choosing entails the risk of eclecticism, incorporating everything while standing for nothing. I was initially drawn to psychoanalytic thinking, because its emphasis on "depth psychology" was intellectually appealing and, I thought addressed the complexity of the human psyche, integrated internal and external forces, and spoke from a developmental perspective. It was my hope that, with enough understanding, arrived at in the right way at the right time in the context of the right therapeutic relationship, people could get better and stay better. But being a psychoanalytic thinker is not simple: are you a Freudian, a Jungian, an Adlerian, a Mahlerian, a Kohutian, an Object Relations therapist or an Ego Psychologist? The choices go on and on.

There was also the hope advanced by cognitive-behavior therapy, with its clearly-delineated techniques and short-term ways of tracking progress that one could actually see and measure improvement. An issue raised by "depth" psychologists was whether the changes using these behavioral techniques were merely "superficial" and did not deal with the "real, underlying issues." But the ability to achieve and recognize short-term gains was appealing to my patients and to me, and particularly helpful with patients coping with medical issues like chronic pain conditions. I was also drawn to family therapy, because of its systems orientation, and to neuro-biological methods, through my training in neurofeedback and biofeedback. So, I thus became a generalist, an eclectic practitioner who tried to learn from everything, integrate it all in my work, and commit myself fully to nothing. Did this make me more flexible, thus better serving my patients? I can't be sure. And did that really matter as long as I applied the techniques, regardless of theoretical orientation, with warmth, empathy and genuineness? Furthermore, was what I considered warmth, empathy and genuineness really what I thought it was?

At one point I sought out private supervision with a well-respected clinician known for his expertise in self-psychology, a school of psychoanalytic theory and technique that emphasizes empathy at its core. I quickly learned that my "empathic" responses were still coming from my own perspective and biases about what was relevant about the patients' experiences, and that, truly entering the patient's reality means understanding and suspending my own, which takes more insight, effort and practice than I had anticipated.

"...I will always look at people and relationships analytically, I will look for the "meaning" behind words and actions, I will examine the antecedents and consequences of behavior and emotion—it is hard letting go of everything that has been part of my professional identity for the past almost fifty years."

Prior to the last several years, the majority of my patients left therapy in a planned manner. We discussed termination and we set a date. This allowed for a process in which whatever gains had been made could be reinforced and solidified, and in which both parties could assess the work and learn from it. Entire trainings were created to deal with this essential developmental process, which was emphasized in the work of the noted psychoanalyst Roy Schaefer. Nowadays, it seems that often people simply leave. They announce their last session during that session, or they just call to cancel or, merely, stop showing up for sessions. This deprives both the patient and the therapist of important opportunities for growth and learning and for taking the time to appreciate and internalize the relationship and its meaning. It's this last phase that helps patients sustain their gains over time. The loss of this last step has made the enterprise of therapy feel much less gratifying to me than it had been previously. I feel it as a great loss.

As I slowly detach myself emotionally from the field (de-cathect, as an analyst might put it), I have decreased my reading of journals and newsletters, and my participation in the several listservs to which I subscribe. I have stopped going to as many trainings as previously, and I have stopped purchasing new testing materials and biofeedback equipment. The field is passing me by, which I find both sad and freeing. Although I will always be a psychologist—I will always look at people and relationships analytically, I will look for the "meaning" behind words and actions, I will examine the antecedents and consequences of behavior and emotion—it is hard letting go of everything that has been part of my professional identity for the past almost fifty years. It is time for me to do other things, set other goals, stop striving to be more/do more/know more in this field and spend my time with other things that are important. It is hard to step out of the road or the river or whatever this is and watch others striving, moving uphill (or upstream), accomplishing good things, and wondering, if only with a bit more practice, I could more fully reach my always just out of reach potential. It is hard to be replaced. It is hard to step aside and wonder: did I matter? And, if I did, will there be a way to still matter?

I hope so, on both fronts.

References

Rogers, C. R. (1951). Client-centered therapy: its current practice, implications, and theory. Boston: Houghton Mifflin.

Szasz, T. S. (1974). The myth of mental illness: foundations of a theory of personal conduct. New York: Harper & Row.

Winnicott, D. W. 1. (1971). Therapeutic consultations in child psychiatry. New York, Basic Books.

David S. Ribner

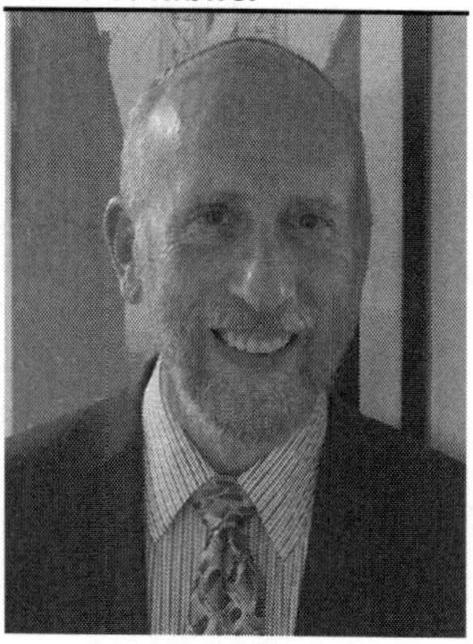

DAVID S. RIBNER earned his BA, Smicha (Rabbinic Ordination), MS (history) and MSW degree from Yeshiva University and his doctorate from Columbia University. He is the founder of the Sex Therapy Training Program, Bar-Ilan University, Israel and is certified as a sex therapist and supervisor in Israel and the U.S. He is in private practice as a sex and marital therapist in Jerusalem, has authored some 40 articles and book chapters and writes and lectures extensively on cultural sensitivity and sexuality. He is also the co-author of Et Le'ehov (A Time to Love): The Newlywed's Guide to Physical Intimacy and (with Talli Rosenbaum) of Ani L'Dodi, I Am for My Beloved: A Guide to Enhanced Intimacy for Married Couples. *matzeel@hotmail.com*

Healing through Poetry

Introduction

CLIENTS WITH SEXUAL ABUSE HISTORIES PRESENT THERAPISTS WITH MULTIPLE CHALLENGES. As with other therapeutic relationships, creating an atmosphere of trust provides clients with a safe space in which to share their painful narratives. However, the unhealed emotional scars of the abused may cause clients to experience our invited verbalizations as adding to their anguish. In such cases, the written word can serve as a messaging option, allowing for communication to be experienced as one step removed and thus more easily tolerated.

This paper focuses on three women, all with histories of sexual abuse – two while children and one as an adult. Though all three became verbally communicative in the therapy room, all chose, as an element of their processes, to use poetry as a means of expressing searing emotions. While collections of this genre of poetry exist in the published literature (*Survivors in Transition,* undated; *Your Voices,* 2017; Klee, 2021), in this article I will place these poems in the context of each client's relevant history with one common theme: the betrayal of trust.

All identifying information has been significantly modified and I have not censored any of the frank, at times brutal language with which these women expressed themselves. Each poem was given to me to be used at my discretion.

Trust and Betrayal

"For trust not him that hath once broken faith" (Shakespeare, Henry VI, part 3, act 4).

Trust has been defined as the willingness of the one

who trusts to become vulnerable to the one being trusted, presuming that the one being trusted will act in the other's best interests (Schilke, Reimann and Cook 2021). Simpson (2007, p.587) has noted that "Trust is one of the most important components—and perhaps the most essential ingredient—for the development and maintenance of happy, well-functioning relationships." Among those who have sought to list the elements of trust within family constellations, a consensus of basic requirements has emerged. A representative listing is provided by Pace (2023): communication, reliability, transparency, vulnerability, accountability, empathy and shared values.

In light of the narratives of these three women, we would add the additional essential components of trust suggested by Cherry (2023)— the provision of safety and security. In these scenarios, various family members, intentionally or not, created or contributed to atmospheres fraught with fear and danger with the most damaging consequence being betrayal of trust.

Each of these women conveyed a clear sense of feeling betrayed; implicit assumptions and expectations about trust in a family context proved to be spurious. In that context, none saw other family members as a potential source of help or safety. Schafer (2021) notes that only trusted people can betray. The intensity of the relationship determines the intensity of the emotional stress caused by the betrayal. Examining the consequences of such betrayal, Freyd (1994) coined the term "betrayal trauma" which describes the powerful emotions described in these poems. "Betrayal trauma" may become a haunting echo played out in subsequent relationships, with "the deepening conviction that relationships can neither be enjoyed, trusted nor expected to last" (Allender, 1990).

In the relationships in which their abuse occurred, these women seemed to have no warning as to the potential for emotional distress and damage. In each case, the perpetrator was a relative, by birth or by marriage, who was initially assumed to present no possibility of risk. Gobin and Freyd (2014) discuss a *tendency to trust,* which describes the expectations of the authors of this poetry. This perhaps makes the betrayal all the more hurtful, since trust was assumed in each situation.

From these case histories and poetry samples, it appears evident that perpetrators did not seek to abuse; rather each sought to slake his own desires, with no consideration for the price paid by the victim. Chan (2009) categorizes this as *incidental betrayal* in contrast with *intentional betrayal.* The former occurs when the abuser violates trust expectations while pursuing other aims, the latter is when the goal of the abuser is to intentionally violate trust expectations.

The consequences of betrayal played out differently in the lives of each of these women. For two, an achieved goal of treatment was to help them differentiate between the men who were abusers and other men who were not, for the third, the outcome was more ambiguous.

The literature addressing interventions for healing the betrayal of trust tends to focus on: 1) re-establishing a positive, healing relationship between the betrayed party and the one seen as the instigator of the betrayal, or 2) working toward enabling any trust once again. As will be seen from their poetry, not one of these three women indicated option 1 as a goal, the emotional scars they carried negated any desire to reconnect with their abusers.

Rehabilitating the ability to trust has been the subject of many sources in professional and popular literature. Reed and Enright (2006) describe a brief therapy model for post relationship, postcrisis (sic) treatment which focuses on anger validation, mourning of losses from the abuse, assertive limit-setting and interpersonal skill building. Kai-Keating, M, Sorsoli, L. and Grossman, F.K. (2010) report the following mechanisms associated with positive adaptation: engaging in safe relationships, gaining a communal and shared sense of belonging, using boundaries to manage relationships, controlling anger, developing intimacy and achieving acceptance. In a third example, Flasch, Murray and Crowe (2015) differentiated between intrapersonal processes and interpersonal processes. Examples of the former included regaining and recreating one's identity, healing from the symptoms of abuse, education and examination of abusive relationships, and acceptance and forgiveness of self and abuser. The latter consisted of two themes: building positive social support and relationships, and using one's experiences to help others,

The popular literature offers almost limitless sources of advice to help the healing process after abuse. Here are some of those sources, with full citations in the bibliography: Wong (2015), Ertel (2022), Smith (2018), Akin (2023), and Wozny (2022).

The clients and their poems

These cases are presented in order of their dates in treatment.

Aviva

Aviva presented as a 23-year-old woman, married three years, with a child 11/2 years old. She, British now living in Israel, and her husband, Dan, from north Africa, grew up in Ultra-Orthodox Jewish families and both were committed to that lifestyle. She described her mother as the dominant parent, who invested considerable time and energy in her children, but who failed to create any real emotional bond with them. Her father, a successful businessman, filled the role of the emotionally available parent.

Aviva's primary presenting problem was a lack of desire to be sexually involved with Dan. Following strict religious dicta, neither she nor her husband had any pre-marital partnered sexual experience. Further, neither had any physical contact at all with any member of the opposite sex, with the exception of direct relatives. Aviva found her husband attractive, "he has a cute body," and would enthusiastically touch him anywhere except his penis, which she described as "repulsive." Nevertheless, she attempted to make herself available to him sexually, which she tolerated by detaching emotionally from the experience. Aviva reported enjoying being naked together, engaging in extensive mutual, non-genital touch. Aviva recounted masturbating to orgasm, without guilt feelings, for as long as she could remember, and always in a prone position. She did not keep this from her husband but would not masturbate in his presence.

Dan was uncomfortable in therapy, particularly with discussing intimate issues in front of a stranger, and by joint agreement, Aviva continued individual sessions, with Dan consenting to return when invited or to be accessible by phone.

In her initial session, I had asked Aviva about any painful memories of her life prior to marriage. After several weeks, Aviva returned to say that she had begun to remember events from her pre-teen years, which she had never consciously experienced as problematic or influential until being asked in therapy. Three months passed before Aviva could speak of these memories in detail or with more than a dismissive attitude. However, an additional mode of communication was available for therapeutic use.

Upon graduating high school, Aviva had informed her parents of her desire to attend college, she graduated with honors and decided on furthering her education with a graduate degree in creative writing. At the start of her therapy, she had begun the second of three semesters, completing the program shortly before ending treatment.

When memories of early sexual trauma began to emerge during our sessions, Aviva struggled with articulating her ever more painful emotional state. My suggestion that she use her writing talents as a means of expression was received skeptically at first, but after her initial attempt, provided a safe outlet for her and valuable therapeutic material, Aviva would periodically e-mail written material, poetry or prose, several days before our sessions. This paper will present examples of her poetry.

Aviva's story, sadly familiar, starts with memories of a loving, affectionate father who gave his children massages. She recalls nothing untoward until age ten or so when he started coming to her room some nights, closing the door, sitting on her bed, and asking her to point her buttocks toward him, take off her panties and then rub his penis against her. This was, he said, because he loved her so much, but she must always keep it their secret. Aviva has no memories of penetration or ejaculation. Her father continued being affectionate in other ways, including massaging her back and chest. Aviva began to feel uncomfortable with this touch when her breasts started developing at age 11. Her father would stop these activities when he thought her mother was approaching Aviva's room, increasing Aviva's uneasiness. Sometime during her twelfth year, she told her father to stop and he did.

Aviva states that not until viewing these events from an adult perspective did she see them as devastating; the physical sensations were at best, warm and comforting, at worst, not unpleasant. She always loved her father and still does. She is more hurt by his having done this to her than by what he actually did. This sense of betrayal, and its impact on her, comprise the basis for much of Aviva's initial written material:

That's why he touched you
The way you never told him to
Where it was cold
On daddy's bed
Under daddy's arms
In between his legs

And pushed down his pants
And his love against you
Into you
Shifting
Pushing
Breathing
Throbbing

That's why he bought you
A red bicycle
And a porcelain doll
That never cried
Little girl
Be happy
Daddy loves you

And he also bought you ice cream
And gumballs
And stickers
And he also bought you earrings
And sunglasses
And headphones
And he also brought you into his bed

The one you always shared
When mom didn't see
And closed the door
And locked it

Be happy
Little girl
Daddy loves you

He loves you
Like he loves himself

In contrast, the following excerpt is taken from a longer letter Aviva was asked to write as part of the therapy termination process. Directed at her father, the decision as to whether to send it was left in her hands; by the end of therapy, it had not been sent:

Fuck you.
That's a new word I learnt in the big, bad secular world,
and I think it describes what you did to me...
You always promised me that I was your favorite daughter
and that you loved me so much.
But you lied.
\you loved only yourself.
Yourself and your penis...
...I loved you so much, my favorite Abbah (father) who turned me into a corpse so when I got married that's what I was.
And still am.
And always will be...
I need a new body...
I need a new mind...
I need a new father...
So I can be a woman.
So I can be normal
So I can love.
So I can have sex...
I obeyed everything you told me...
But then I got married and they told me nothing
But we figured out something—together
That what my husband does to me as a man
You did to me as a father.
When a dad acts like a man to a daughter
He is a murderer, a murderer, a murderer.
And I want to ask you
My father who is a murderer,
One question—which will never be answered
A question—which will never be asked
A question—I live with, I sleep with, I'll die with...
Why?

Beth

Beth and her husband Efram, both in their late 20's, entered couples treatment with complaints of general marital dissatisfaction. Sexual incompatibility soon became a therapy focus, primarily for Efram, complaining of a lack of sexual satisfaction and lack of interest on Beth's part. From her perspective, Beth described Efram as an insensitive and uncaring lover.

At the start of therapy they had been married 7 years, with one child. Both were born and raised in Australia in more liberal religious families and had met during university studies. Soon after their wedding they had moved to Israel, a plan agreeable to both.

A good poem distills and enlarges reality at the same time.

—Christian Wiman

On paper, this seemed to be an ideal match. Efram, an actuary, grew up in an intact, two parent family, with each child raised with high expectations of academic and professional accomplishment. He had found employment in a respected firm, but felt his work standards were not sufficiently appreciated by his managers.

Beth described her intact family as warm and supportive. She had earned a degree as a physical therapist, but found her career path doing medical research in Israel. She saw parenting as a primary focus of her time and energy.

Beth and Efram had begun dating during their university days, but by mutual religious conviction, there was no physical contact until after their wedding ceremony. Each denied any partnered pre-marital sexual activity, with Beth acknowledging a history of guilt-free masturbation starting during early childhood, primarily as a way of relaxing at bedtime.

Efram was always a reluctant participant in therapy and about a year after beginning our contact, he left therapy while Beth continued. This change allowed Beth the opportunity to speak much more freely, to become aware of normative physical and emotional intimacy and then to begin describing a sexually and emotionally abusive marital relationship. The couple separated after 8 years of marriage and divorced a year later.

Beth's sexual victimization began on her wedding night. She remembers being forced by Efram to have intercourse while she was asleep, awakening to intense vaginal pain. Lacking adequate sexual information, and without previous sexual contacts, Beth was unsure if this was the experience of every virgin's first-time intercourse. Efram's sexual demands continued during most of the years the couple lived together. In the course of therapy, both with Efram and individually, Beth gradually became aware of the extent of her lack of accurate sexual information and consequently, the extent of her sexual victimization.

At one point, Beth wrote a manifesto for herself detailing the sexual abuse she suffered. It begins, "Efram, following are the ways in which you chose to degrade women over a period of eight years. You chose to:" Beth then lists twelve illustrations of this abuse, including the following examples:

- ...the only way a woman could demonstrate her love for you, and thereby receive your "love" was to yield her vagina to your service.
- Laugh at a woman's intimacy when she attempted to minister to your needs.
- Touch a woman's intimate parts after she requested that you desist. This in order to arouse in her a desire to serve you.
- Humiliate a woman by demanding she lay flat on her back in other people's homes where thin walls would advertise your dominance over her to the home's inhabitants.
- Require a woman to explain herself when she voiced a preference against your choice of sexual position... then to question her right to such choices and inclinations.

Beth ended the manifesto with this: "In the event that you wish to further engage in heterosexual physical intimacy, it behooves you to acquire a degree of respect for your woman counterpart. In the absence of that, one word: castrate."

Toward the end of Beth's weekly individual sessions, at her request, we revisited her recollections of her wedding night in a hotel room, which she could now, almost a decade later, view as a better informed and more self-aware divorced woman. Several weeks afterwards, Beth brought this poem to our session. Sending this to Efram would have meant creating a connection to him, an option she wished to avoid at all costs.

You fucked me in my sleep
on our wedding night,
after ramming your long-petrified cock
into a center I did not know how to yield.
The sound and feel, I recall.
Not the smell.
My eyes were shut.
My screams, as you struck,
were loud.
My tears scorched hotter cheeks.
When you could not enter,
You lay, a sweaty haired ape, beside me.
You had not showered.
Did you lull me then to sleep,
or, hunched, wait for your prey?
Did you plunge as my breath quieted?
Or did you stay to watch my breath quiet
As I slept?
I woke to the pain of splitting apart,
and to you rising
to sleep on cleaner sheets
in a fresher bed.

Deborah

By the time Deborah was twenty years old, she was already divorced. Married at nineteen against her will through a match parentally arranged, Deborah stayed with her husband for three weeks, before leaving and establishing herself independently in another country. Their marriage was never consummated. Deborah refused any physical contact with her husband. Despite efforts of parents and counselors to bring this couple back together, they were divorced after a year.

During the period of her separation from her husband, Deborah entered treatment with a desire to understand her marriage. A primary motivation was the hope of another marriage, with a much more positive outcome. Deborah remained in treatment for a year, worked with special needs children to support herself, and shared an apartment with three other women.

In her family-of-origin narrative, Deborah described a conservative, rigidly religious upbringing in which she felt entirely comfortable and with no thoughts of altering this belief system for herself. She saw her family as functional, but she recalled few expressions of physical affection. While Deborah's arranged marriage was consistent with the values and expectations of her community, this was the point at which she felt abandoned by her family. She had not wished to be married, not to this man or to any man, and she vividly recalled her strong objections falling on deaf ears.

This issue became the initial focus of treatment, involving topics of empowerment, family and community ties, reality testing and decision making, among others. As the therapy progressed, Deborah began to express a profound aversion to any possibility of mutual physical touch with a man. She denied any sexual desire for women, had no experience with masturbation (she did not know what it was) and denied any history of sexual abuse or harassment. Consistent with her background, Deborah had minimal sexual information or body awareness.

Due to the intensity of her sexual aversion, we returned several times to explore the possibility of an unremembered sexual trauma. During one session, I went through a list with her of various relatives with whom the family had contact. When the word "uncle" was used, Deborah began to shake and cry, in contrast to her usual presentation of poise, manners and control.

Starting with a vague recollection, Deborah told of an episode with an uncle when she was ten or eleven years old. This man, a bachelor, had stayed with her family during a time when he was adrift in his life. Deborah remembered that she awoke one night to see this uncle in her bedroom. When he saw that she was awake, he dropped his pants and showed her his penis, which she describes as "huge and purple." She had no memory of any physical touch and is fairly certain that this happened only once. She had never told anyone, and had repressed this memory until it arose during this session.

For several years, Deborah had been keeping a journal in which she recorded feelings, impressions and experiences. She hid the notebooks in her room and showed them to no one. Several months after we had begun to process this sexual trauma, Deborah offered to share three poems she had written about this newly recalled event. The poems are lengthy and I have included here excerpts from one of them, written to her uncle, but not sent. Words in parentheses are English translations from the original Hebrew.

You've ruined me to great lengths and heights
You've trapped me in coarse ropes and ties
You've turned round to move on with life
Ignoring my heart wrenching, silent cries

You've stripped me you've sliced through my heart
You've invaded, intruded my very private part
You've allowed your desires to control
Leaving a wide, gaping, bottomless hole

The selfishness and roughness you've shown
You thought you're in charge – I'm your own
You've treated me like rubbish picked directly from the bin
You forgot I have a heart within my skin

Oh how I wish I could pay back
But the resources and powers I lack
And I don't wish to initiate strife
I'll have zero pleasure to have ruined your life

The Missing Curative Element

My work with these women incorporated some of the guidelines mentioned in the first section of this paper, but arguably the most significant healing component finds scant citation in the professional literature, namely the therapeutic relationship. Various authors have contributed descriptions and analyses of therapeutic relationships [e.g. Hill and Knox (2009), Chowdhury (2006), Beutler and Harwood (2002), Scourteli and Lennie (2011)]. In the cases analyzed here, the developed therapeutic relationship with these women included the following elements:

Boundaries—the violation of expected, normative boundaries characterized these abusive situations, thus maintaining the safety of clear boundaries in the therapy room was essential. Establishing and maintaining these boundaries included an agreed upon contract, clarifying informed consent, time management, and judiciously limiting therapist self-disclosure.

Respect—as these women felt a pervasive lack of respect in their abusive relationships, it was imperative that they feel respected in this therapeutic relationship. One aspect was seeing each of them as complete human beings and not only the elements of their symptoms or traumatizing histories. Respect was also manifest in underscoring their exclusive control over anything they wished to convey during the sessions.

Empathy—elements of empathy in a therapeutic relationship included attempts at careful listening, conveying understanding, accepting the other's experiences and perceptions and connecting to the other's personal distress. The task of empathy was both cognitive and emotional, seeking to perceive and process each client's world through that client's eyes. Successful use of empathy required that these women felt nonjudgmentally accepted throughout the therapy experience.

Confronting abuse—although never entirely comfortable, each of these women became capable of describing and then confronting their abuse histories. When necessary and appropriate, they made use of poetry to give dramatic expression to their profound traumatic experiences. The challenge was to modulate each narrative in order to prevent, as much as possible, the addition of further layers of emotional scar tissue.

The elements listed above—boundaries, respect, empathy—came into play at various stages of the developing therapeutic relationship, allowing for at least a partial healing process unique to each woman. As with many therapeutic experiences, this work, for all participants, had moments of frustration, doubts, fears, hesitation and tears. The more positive aspects included relief, understanding, acceptance, renewal and perhaps more importantly, hope for the future.

The Therapist

In discussing the other "partner" involved in the therapeutic relationship, one factor must be acknowledged at the outset—I am a male therapist, of the same gender as the abusers of these victims. Upon reflection, I would not advocate such a referral, since an initial contact with a female therapist may afford greater comfort and security. These

> "Each of these women conveyed a clear sense of feeling betrayed; implicit assumptions and expectations about trust in a family context proved to be spurious."

three women began their work with me with a marital issue as the presenting problem, their abuse experiences later revealed gradually during the course of our sessions.

Because of the volatility and anguish of their narratives, empathy could easily have evolved into sympathy, with minimal therapeutic value. I have previously worked with abused clients, yet in these instances the poetry provided a different lens through which to view the reality of their wounding relationships. I had no prior experience regarding this poetic aspect of the treatment process nor was I able to discover any relevant literature or consult with colleagues who had done parallel work. I chose to proceed with each woman, exploring their poetry with the goal of helping them find, where possible, relevance and meaning for their lives, past and present. The awareness and appropriate responses required to manage this process proved unexpectedly challenging for me.

It soon became evident that a constant preoccupation with this written material during each session had the risk of becoming emotionally draining and counterproductive for all involved. However, as we gradually explored the lines of poetry, the women became more comfortable with connecting the text to their narratives. It is beyond my expertise to do a word-by-word textual analysis of this written material, and I attempted to maintain our focus on the evoked emotions.

As with many of our cases, and as described above, endings were determined more by circumstance than by contract. Upon reflection, I do not stake any claim as to a new therapy model or intervention—there will be no marketing of a revolutionary three stage training program. Any accomplishment was the result of doing what most of us do, namely making the best use of the material entrusted to us by our clients, mindful of the necessary elements of a therapeutic relationship and open to the new and unexpected. I had never before considered poetry as clinical raw material, and its use is what I share with you in this paper.

Bibliography

Akin, E, (2023). 10 ways to trust yourself after narcissistic abuse, *Unfilteredd* (sic), unfilteredd.net/10-ways-to-trust-yourself-after-experiencing-narcissistic-abuse/

Allender, D. (1990). *The wounded heart,* Nav Press, Carol Stream, IL p. 121.

Beutler, L.F. and Harwood, T.M. (2002). What is and can be attributed to the therapeutic relationship? *Journal of Contemporary Psychotherapy,* 32(1), 25-33.

Chan, M. E. (2009). "Why did You Hurt Me?" Victim's Interpersonal Betrayal Attribution and Trust Implications. *Review of General Psychology,* 13(3), 262-274.

Cherry, K. (2023). Why you may have trust issues and how to overcome them. *Very Well Mind,* www.verywellmind.com – 5215390.

Chowdhury, S,R, (2006), How is the therapeutic relationship talked into being? *Journal of Family Therapy,* 28(2), 153-174.

Ertel, A, (2022). How to heal from emotional abuse. *Talkspace,* www.talkspace.com/blog/healing-after-emotional-abuse/.

Flasch, P., Murray, C.E. &and Crowe, A. (2015). Overcoming abuse: A phenomenological investigation of the journey to recovery from past intimate partner violence. *Journal of Interpersonal Violence,* 32(22), 3373-3401.

Freyd, J.J. (1994) Betrayal-trauma: Traumatic amnesia as an adaptive response to childhood abuse. *Ethics & Behavior,* 4, 307-329.

Gobin, R.L. & Freyd, J.J. (2014). The impact of betrayal trauma on the tendency to trust. *Psychological Trauma: Theory, Research, Practice, and Policy,* 6(5), 505–511.

Hill, C.E. and Knox, S. (2009). Processing the therapeutic relationship, *Psychotherapy Research,* 19(1), 13-29.

Kai-Keating, M., Sorsoli, L. & Grossman, F.K. (2010). Relational challenges and recovery processes in male survivorsof childhood sexual abuse. *Journal of Interpersonal Violence,* 25(4), 666-683.

Klee, A. (2021). Unhomed: A collection of poems about surviving after rape, independently published.

Pace, R. (2023). 7 elements of trust: The foundation of a strong relationship, *Marriage.com.*

Reed, G.L & Enright, R.D. (2006). The effects of forgiveness therapy on depression, anxiety, and posttraumic stress for women after spousal emotional abuse, *Journal of Counseling and Clinical Psychology,* 74(5), 920-929.

Schafer, J. (2021). Betrayal and human relationships, *Psychology Today,* https://www.psychologytoday.com/intl/blog/let-their-words-do-the-talking/202111/betrayal-and-human-relationships

Schilke, O, Reimann, M. & Cook, K.S. (2021). Trust in social relationships, *Annual Review of Sociology,* 47, 239-259.

Scourteli, M.C. and Lennie, C. (2011). The therapeutic relationship from an attachment theory perspective, *Counselling Psychology Review,* 26(1), 20-33.

Simpson, J.A. (2007). Foundations of interpersonal trust in *Social psychology: Handbook of basic principles,* chap.25, Academia.edu.

Smith, E.-M. (2018). Trusting again after abuse in a relationship, HealthyPlace, www.healthyplace.com/blogs/verbalabuseinrelationships/2018/04/trusting-again-after-an-abusive-relationship.

Survivors poetry, *Survivors in Transition* (undated), https://survivorsintransition.co.uk/poetry

Wong, B. (2015). 9 Things to know about loving again after emotional abuse. *Huffpost,* www.huffpost.com/entry/what-to-know-about-loving-again-after-emotional-abuse_n_5672fe39e4b0688701dc970a.

Wozny, C. (2022). Learning how to trust yourself after abuse, *Healthyplace.* www.healthyplace.com/blogs/verbalabuseinrelationships/2022/6/learning-how-to-trust-yourself

Your Voices (2017). Sexual Assault Support Services of Midcoast Maine, https://www.sassmm.org/uploads/1/0/1/7/101776612/your_voices_2017.pdf

Of the healing arts, therapy is surely the most literary, since it involves the telling and revision of a story. And of the literary arts, therapy's the oddest and most intimate, because the story is told for one listener only, and that listener becomes a collaborator in the shaping of the tale. No listener is ever asked to work harder, or to take more of a hand in the work of bringing order to the broken pieces of a narrative.

—*Mark Doty, poet*

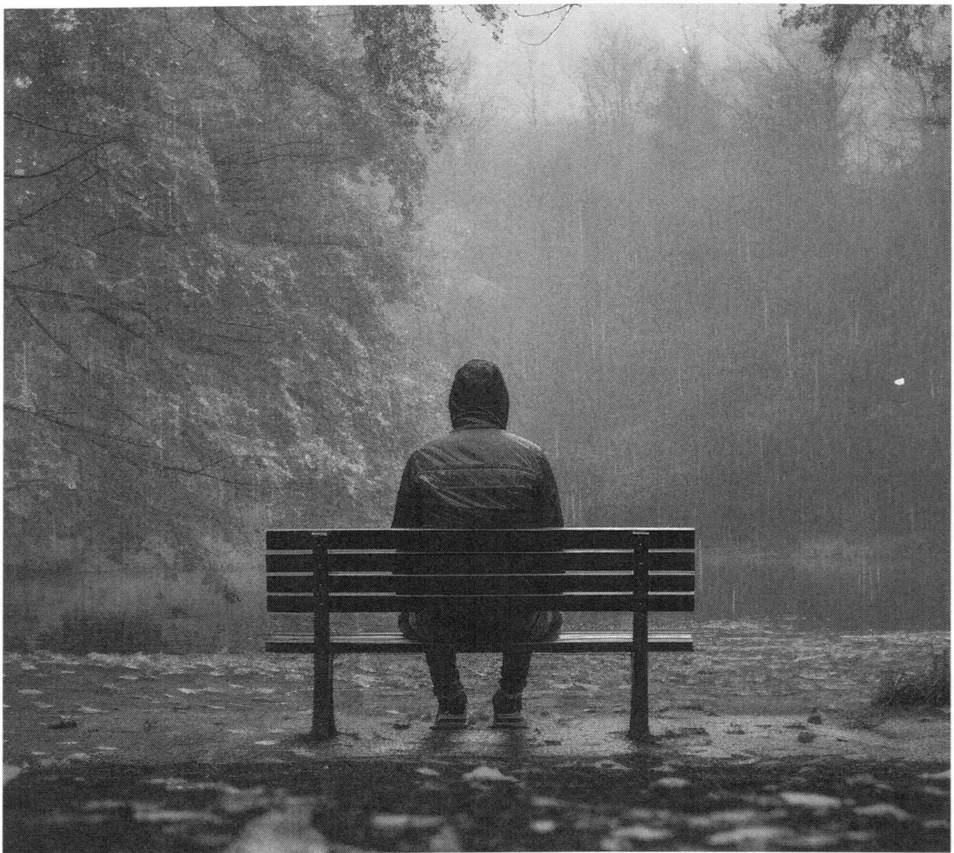

Sitting on a Bench by Iftikhar Alam

Judith Logue

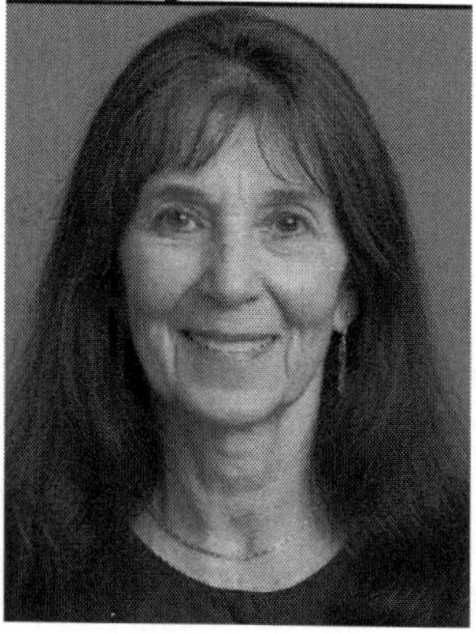

JUDY LOGUE, PHD is a senior psychoanalyst and professional coach in practice for 50 years. Dr Logue is a co-founder of the Institute for Psychoanalysis and Psychotherapy of NJ, a former board member of two divisions of the American Psychological Association (APA), past Director at Large, and current Alternate Director on the American Psychoanalytic Association (APsA) BOD. She publishes book reviews, book chapters, and papers in professional journals. You may reach her at *judith@judithlogue.com*; 609-915-9155.

Treating a Dying Patient—
Flying the Plane and "The New Horizon"

THIS CHRONICLE IS ABOUT THE FINAL STAGE OF TREATMENT OF A MAN WITH METASTATIC PROSTATE BONE CANCER, WHOM I CALL "MICHAEL." He died in 2018. This paper is gratefully dedicated to him.

The treatment of Michael was a catalyst for my own interest in the topic of death, stirring many feelings and promoting a deeper understanding of some of the theories about death and treatment techniques, and about myself—how I think and feel about death and how it relates to my earlier history.

What I am presenting is the story of our struggle. Little of it was conscious until later. I learned—and am still learning—about my own and others' varied reactions to death, I know well that the fear of death is a common fear, although impairment and disability are usually our worst fears. I can often imagine death, and I have seen it. However, constant worry about death and dying is a psychological problem; a preoccupation with the fear of dying may be the fear of living.

Sudden or slow, death and dying are highly personal—and experienced in so many individual ways. I hope my perspective will be a catalyst for your own theories, thoughts and feelings. Ideally, it might also increase awareness of any countertransference responses you may encounter in a clinical situation.

Some Personal History Related to Death

Like many of the people I know, I have thought deeply about death for a long time. At age 9, I carried on and insisted that I be allowed to attend Grandpop's funeral, wanting to satisfy my curiosity about death, and most importantly, to get my wish to say goodbye. My mother defied convention by allowing me to go, as children were not supposed to go to funerals. Mother also allowed me to kiss my beloved grandfather goodbye in the open casket. This was a tender moment, and this introduction to death has forever helped me cope with grief and upset when I lose a person I love.

I realized that at least I don't deny death, though I am often afraid of it—especially the probability of physical decline, disability, and grueling medical and hospice care, as happened to my patient Michael. Humor helps me a lot, so I joke with trusted friends that I plan to die at 102, dreaming about sex and airplanes. My peers who are age 80 to 100 send regular jokes about aging to help us with our "organ recitals" and what we call, "The Medical Mill." Judy Viorst's book, Making the Best of What's Left: When We're Too Old to Get the Chairs Reupholstered, speaks to me! I have few illusions about immortality. I do not have an interest in dedicating my life to achieving a legacy to change the world, or for fame. I just hope to be a better person today than I was yesterday and a better person tomorrow than today. However, in writing this paper about treating Michael, to my surprise, I discovered that not everything is settled for me when it comes to dying and death.

Psychotherapy and Death

I became anxious when I realized that I was going to share the treatment of Michael with colleagues. I started reading books, exploring theories, and different models and techniques for treatment. Intellectualization usually calms me. It adds insight and understanding to my emotional reactions.

Elisabeth Kubler-Ross, a Swiss American psychiatrist and pioneer, wrote a groundbreaking book, On Death and Dying (1969) that presents a theory of the five states of grief known as the "Kubler-Ross Model." That model seemed ridiculous to me until I discovered that she believes the stages are not linear and do not progress in a predictable way. Michael even brought up Kubler-Ross during our therapy as we raced to the finish line.

Treating a Dying Patient—The Case of Michael

Michael is very different from the patient of Dr. Judy Kantrowitz who discussed death in Reflections on Mortality: A Patient Faces Death, which appeared in the Journal of the American Psychoanalytic Association in 2017. Her patient suffered emotionally and with great psychological pain.

Dr. Kantrowitz' analysand, a 60-year-old woman, experienced an identity crisis—going from a tireless high- functioner to an exhausted, weakened, dependent person who no longer recognized herself. She was highly articulate about her emotions, her self-sacrificing, depressive proclivities, and her overwhelming fears about dying.

In contrast, Michael insisted on "flying the plane to the ground," like Sully -- the airline pilot who landed his plane in the Hudson River. Michael wanted to function at his best as a father of sons, a husband, and a patient. Action and functioning took precedence. Introspection and talking about feelings were important, but less so than activities of daily living and leaving a legacy for his wife and sons.

Understanding how each case of dying is unique was helpful to me.

Some Background

Michael was a 60-year-old, white, married father of highly intelligent 20-year-old twin sons. He was well educated and worked as a landscape architect, working for several companies for twenty years.

At age 47, in 2002, Michael was referred to me by a friend of his wife, for anxiety issues. Michael saw me for weekly psychotherapy until 2006. He then returned for therapy in 2013, after a 7-year hiatus. A year later, in 2014, Michael was diagnosed with Stage IV prostate cancer. The cancer had metastasized to his bones. He died a few years later on March 15, 2018.

Because I had moved from NJ to a Florida airport community in 2012, we met by Skype. Until 2015, we also met every 1-3 months in a colleague's NJ office. Our mutual aviation interest was a critical aspect of the transference and countertransference issues.

Initially, Michael had thought his high PSA—prostate-specific antigen—level was just something to be watched. With no health insurance, a very low family income, and college-bound sons, he had put off his own health care. Because she could make a better income, his wife worked outside the home. He worked inside the home and had become the primary parent, starting when his twin boys were five years old. He was a devoted husband and loved to teach. When one of his sons had trouble adjusting to middle school, Michael home-schooled him. Because of the constant threat of bankruptcy, I treated Michael pro bono for the last 3 and a half years post-diagnosis.

Michael was a highly intelligent man who functioned at a normal-neurotic level. He was sensitive, at times emotionally reactive or demanding, and used intellectualization as a defense. He had a delightful sense of humor. His awareness of absurdity, irony, people, and social and cultural dynamics enhanced his upset and anger at injustice and un-intelligent behaviors. Michael had a punitive superego which was usually overactive and was among his most intractable traits that therapy and life did little to modify.

Case Overview—Flying the Plane

Michael's request that we write about him came out of the blue, the first week of February 2018, 6 weeks before he died. I met Michael and his wife for couple visits in 2011 for two years. His wife expressed gratitude and relief that he trusted and felt helped by me, and she was the one who suggested we write about this.

Michael and I agreed on co-authorship of a presentation, with much back and forth about confidentiality and journal publication issues. Michael asked me to do two things. First, observe what he had done in what he called "attempting to fly the plane." Second, to make some professional judgment about how well he had done that.

My own analysis of my ambivalence about this case write-up came to mind months later: maybe it was the coincidental call for papers for a conference with a deadline of March 10th.; maybe this was a way to work through my own feelings about my own life-threatening cancer in 2008, and my own fears about death; maybe both pathological and healthy narcissism; maybe my wish not to be abandoned by Michael and write about him on my own; maybe a mutual wish for immortality. Perhaps all the above and more.

We started writing together in the first week of February 2018, when I told him the submission deadline was March 10th. At that time, he said: "I don't suppose the deadline will allow review of how well things came out in the end, since I intend to outlive the deadline. Maybe you could add that for some later submission elsewhere."

Thinking we were in the home stretch, I wrote the following notes in the first week in March. (These are my actual notes)

"Michael had to cancel the first session ever because he is not well enough. From my perspective, he has been outstanding in flying the plane, keeping up best he can with his medical care (which is brutal beyond description), family obligations whenever possible (and very upsetting to him because he is failing to be able to do them), and being an engaged father and husband. He has always suffered a most severe and punitive superego, is conscientious, reliable and his own worst critic."

I completed editing the conference submission proposal and removal of identifying information on March 8th. Again, from my notes:

"Michael can no longer see me for video sessions and talks briefly when possible. He is trying to preserve energy for a final visit to his wife's family's upstate NY compound with one of his sons."

At the time we did not know he would be gone the following Thursday.

A Title for Our Write-Up? Be Careful What You Ask For

Like process notes, the following excerpts from our email dialogue, with my annotations, offer a window into the last two months of Michael's life. Throughout our online conversation—like the sound of an airplane engine—his impending death roared underneath.

I'll now quote Michael's initial responses to my questions about a working title and how to get started.

Michael wrote: "Be Careful What You Ask For" seemed to pop out as a working title. It just sprang from a moment of SNL (Saturday Night Live) humor.

"During a shared giggle you and I realized what we might have bitten off in the work. This isn't simply because the deadline is so short; but also, because the topic of my dying, my approach to it, appears within the context of a very long, very deep relationship, within which this part is only one chapter that needs, somehow, to be isolated for independent treatment.

"Writing about me will be of value to me. I know, what an ego, right? But I hope, more, that I might be of help to others as well.

"My dying, in fact, isn't even the last chapter, since my deepest hope for whatever I do before I run out of time is that I will leave the deepest possible bonds of joy and love for my family to share in my absence.

"The most important element in our relationship, starting almost from the handshake, is that you never hid behind your professional credentials to avoid our issues. Never any BS; and when you couldn't avoid it, you were the one who warned us we were about to step in it. And, since you have asked before about transference, in my mind, it's just one more moving part in the process of human relationship."

Taking Off—Flying the Plane and the Next Horizons

Next, we had discussions about how best to organize and tell, in Michael's own words, how he thinks and feels about facing death. Michael, understandably, wanted me to take care of him and do all the writing. I refused. We were struggling together with his impending death.

When we discussed titles for writing up Michael's situation, one idea of mine was "The Last Horizon." I thought it was the title of a Memoriam column in my women pilots' magazine. But the actual title is "New Horizons," not "Last Horizons."

Michael reacted strongly; his upset and anger were palpable. He reprimanded me when he told me he did not like the horizon idea. Not only that, but he also told me in his inimitable pedantic style, the word has specific and useful meanings in navigation, meteorology and design.

I defensively explained I had taken it from the 99s magazine column and made a mistake. We ended up in a discussion about the afterlife. With wisecracking - typical of both of us—he set me straight and made me laugh. When I asked him to let me know if there is an afterlife, he gave me a Skype straight-in-the-eye look and said, "Judy, you are not my priority!"

I quickly realized that I was in pain, with my own roiling stages of grief. I struggled with the imminent loss of Michael and was uncertain how I would mourn and master my expectable bereavement. I was trying to accept his death.

Michael's anger at his tragic situation was understandable. But I was angry, too. I did not want to lose him. Perhaps Michael was angry at me for surviving when he would not? Nevertheless, only later was I aware of guilt about surviving my cancer when he could not survive his.

Note that I was unable to interpret our mutual, half-conscious narcissism, distress, pain, sadness and anger that Michael would die soon. I defensively stayed on the surface. We were enacting, in our individual ways, our fears, conflicts and anger about separation, abandonment, and death with a fight about the horizon. Michael is expressive. He was pissed at his situation and at me. I was not at the top of his list for contact from the afterlife!

At the same time, this intensity and helplessness were balanced by the movie about Captain Chesley Sullenberger, which held a compelling theme for Michael. In retrospect, for me as well.

Facing Death: Michael's Defenses for Coping

Michael wrote the following in the third week of February, after we decided to write something:

"Sadly, I have no personal diary of the last three and a half years; so, dates of events and how specific news or treatments affected me are just gone...

"I know I wrote earlier about how the mission of my therapy changed from spouse to spouse/parent, to dying spouse parent. And you and I have talked some about how the last iteration took us off the reservation and out of your expertise. That's part of how the idea for writing me up came to mind. I don't think ANYONE has the expertise to deal with the way I want to deal with all of this.

"And that makes you good for this work. Your candor and wisdom would produce a unique perspective on 'The Case of the Unique Dying Guy.'

"You may remember I didn't have a way to express my goals concisely until I got to see the movie, 'Sully.' In that, Sullenberger's initial flight instructor told him, 'No matter what happens, keep flying the plane.'

"That grabbed me personally.

"Now I have no idea how I've actually handled the stages of grief; though I swear I haven't been able to keep them separate. I started working on acceptance immediately, simply because the other stages seemed like distractions; and it seemed to me that the people I love needed me to face the things, so they'd have more time to.

"The idea of flying the plane has the additional advantage of keeping one busy enough to embrace some optimism. To keep finding things to do; and keep whatever sportsmanship was possible to make things easier for everyone else whenever I had the energy. And not get sidetracked by self-pity or guilt, or anger at any thought someone else could have done more or done better.

"Most of that energy is gone now. I no longer have any control of my affect, no matter what I'm feeling inside. I can laugh on the inside; but I don't remember feeling physically strong enough to laugh out loud.

".... If we're going to add a flying metaphor to the inside joke; then what I've got is a ridge I'm not going to clear between me and my destination airport. And the earth is round. There are no last horizons."

Legacy and Love

In the fourth week of February, Michael writes about his legacy.

"I don't care much how people remember me. Can't control it anyway. Nor do I have a specific wish in memoriam, except that this project might serve some purpose beyond keeping me busy.

"What I want, almost desperately, is for people in my life to continue to have each other in the way I have them now.

"I hope this helps; because I'm so out of ideas."

The Last Communications

Michael's last writing to me in early March is harder to follow than other writing. Some of what he wrote:

- "I feel like Rocky Raccoon from the Beatles song, 'I'll be better as soon as I am able.' I just need a couple of days to get over the beating from yesterday.... I feel like I'm too busy living this way of dying to do more than put one foot in front of the other.
- " .... Every long-term relationship, professional and other, has ups and downs. It's all a single thing to me.
- "I have an instinct. I try to check the action step with trusted resources, chiefly my wife and you, then I try to execute the step itself. To tell the truth in right language, and at the right time for it to be helpful.
- "I apologize if these thoughts are in too raw a state to be of use as is."

"Last thing, since I'm producing more typos than product at this point; I'd love it if the end of this presentation included a prognosis for my family's emotional health after I'm gone, no matter how impossible or simply impossibly vain that wish might be. Those are the horizons that matter to me."

Closing Note

In the last week of February, I wrote that I was still "too much in the experience for objectivity and distance," but that I thought Michael had succeeded in his treatment goals and as many life goals as possible. I said to him, "you have been saying goodbye and doing everything you can to tell everyone what you feel, think and want."

Michael did life review with me, and separately with his wife and sons. Referring to Erikson's model in Childhood and Society for the last stage of life, Michael achieved wisdom during despair. It is hard for me to imagine anyone in these circumstances "flying the plane" better.

I viewed Michael's Sully metaphor as emblematic of the kind of person he was. Michael's approach to death was not "the last horizon" of my unconscious slip. But it was "a new horizon" in the way he was dying. Michael was protective of his family; he was living an active life as much as he could. He willed himself to see that his plight—and his flight—toward death was not a last horizon, but rather a new horizon with the love and protection of his family.

We both wished Michael's finale could have matched Sully's, and in some ways it did. There was no crash landing and the passengers of Michael's life—his family—loved him, just as the passengers of US Airways Flight 1549 were grateful to their pilot, Chesley Sullenberger. Implicit in my relationship with him were my love and respect, as well.

His identification with me is also an aspect of Michael's transference—especially since my move to Florida had a profound effect on how we could continue his psychotherapy.

Over the years, Michael analyzed both positive and negative projections. He also expressed valid criticism, with appropriate anger or superego rage, when I misunderstood, or was clueless about, what he was trying to tell me or figure out.

In the years since Michael's death, I have had time and distance to think about transference and countertransference issues. Michael was more of a gift than a burden, but still a difficult responsibility.

When Michael first asked me to present his case to colleagues, I refused. Selfishly, it seemed like too much work, when I felt I had already given enough. I'm pleased to report that Michael's wish to contribute to my education and learning, if not to others, has been effective - more than I imagined. No matter how much experience one has as a clinician, we always have something new and difficult to address and learn. One is rarely, if ever, immune to entanglements and enactments.

At the same time, being with Michael at the end of his life—and most important—being able to be of some use to him and his family, has been a reward greater than any fee.

My engagement was authentic. I did not feel sorry for Michael—and he did not feel sorry for himself. I felt sorry life and circumstances were cruel—and are for all of us at times. I loved and respected Michael, and I trusted him to be his best self.

I learned that even in this age of "scientism," it is essential to have and to integrate heart, soul and love.

Mentoring Moments

In this section, you will find brief, first-person accounts of memorable encounters with mentors or colleagues that added links to the chain of personal accumulated psychotherapeutic wisdom. We looked for experiences that contained a valuable nugget about the work and the process of becoming a psychotherapist. We are pleased to share these small but powerful gems.

—Hallie Lovett

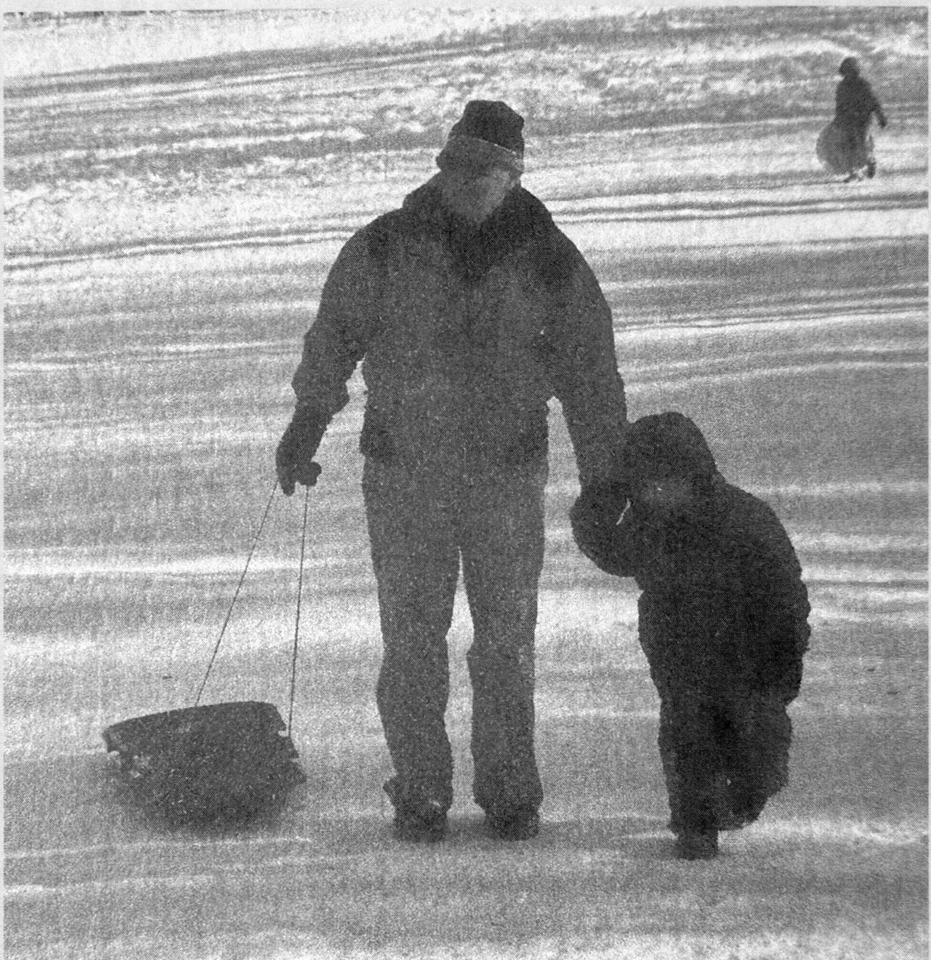

Links in the Chain by Molly Donovan

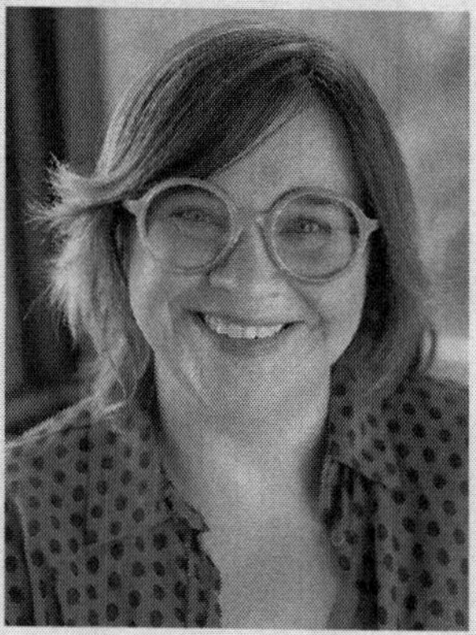

Turtles

by Campbell States, LICSW

I WORKED AT A VERY ROUGH DRUG AND ALCOHOL CLINIC IN A VERY ROUGH PART OF TOWN MY FIRST YEAR OUT OF GRADUATE SCHOOL. Our patients regularly sold drugs outside and carried weapons inside the clinic. I didn't know how to do therapy. I didn't know how to do therapy in a place where patients who had a full set of teeth one week appeared the following week with every tooth removed and no explanation.

If therapy is a process of making sense together, what do you do in a world of utter nonsense? I ran a three-hour intensive outpatient (IOP) group twice a week with another newbie therapist. We asked the clinic director what exactly we should be doing in this group. He advised "don't let them take a smoke break for more than 15 minutes because that's Medicaid fraud." He had no comment about the remaining two hours and forty-five minutes.

"Our patients regularly sold drugs outside and carried weapons inside the clinic."

Lacking sensible guidance from my superiors, I sought outside consultation from Annie, a cheerful almost retired LCSW from the local clinical social work society. Annie had always wanted to be a zoologist, but her gender and circumstance made social work the only viable career path. She was warm and inviting with a house full of pets. Her new puppy Gabe joined us at every meeting. He was a menace but knew the right moment to snuggle up with me when I was distraught. Annie could never remember if we were meeting for 45 minutes or 90 minutes so our sessions had a random cadence. Sometimes she would forget all together. She unfailingly asked me if I wanted to take home a baby turtle from her tank. I never did, but it felt like she was offering a piece of herself to travel with me through frightening waters.

In a wild and boundaryless work situation she showed me that the rules I had been taught in school wouldn't always be there to steady me. but authenticity and the relationship would hold me.

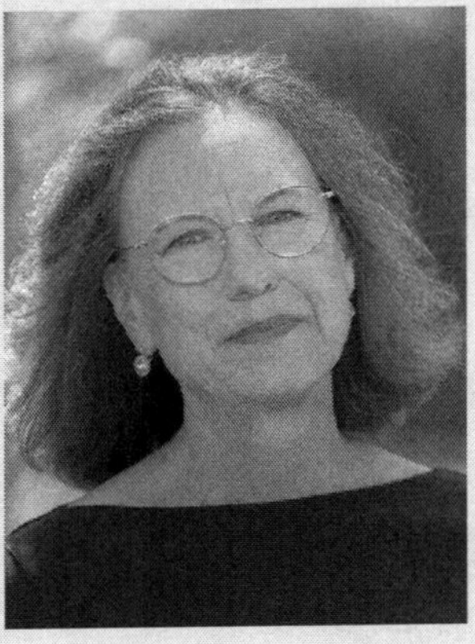

By the Way
by Penelope Norton, PhD

IN THE EARLY 80S I WAS A NEWLY GRADUATED PHD WORKING IN AN AGENCY IN BOCA RATON, FLORIDA. I had relocated there after graduate school in Rochester, New York. After a one year post doc, I joined a mental health charity. I was providing group and individual therapy and supervising graduate students.

Throughout my grad school years, as well as in my post doc, I had maintained my focus on services for children and families. I had evolved from my teen days as a babysitter, college days as an au pair, and as a mentee of a child and developmental psychology professor at University of Florida.

> "I have never forgotten Gene's words from almost forty years ago."

While working in Boca Raton I had a chance social encounter with Gene Shapiro, formally (A. Eugene Shapiro, PhD), a tanned athletic guy who fit the description as a Florida retiree golfer, but who was a highly esteemed recipient of an APA Award for Distinguished Service, from his lifelong psychology practice.

He was newly retired, with a small private practice and a burgeoning role at Nova Southeastern University's Psy.D. program. We briefly chatted, and I shared with him that my focus was on kids and families. He said, "I used to do that, too, and then I realized how all those years spent working with kids uniquely trained me to understand the childhood experiences of the adults who sought therapy; and, as I aged, I transitioned to seeing adults."

I am older now than he was then, and though I still see a few children, I delight in the now finely honed lens through which I see my adult clients. I have never forgotten Gene's words from almost forty years ago, nor his impromptu field guide to my own evolution as a therapist.

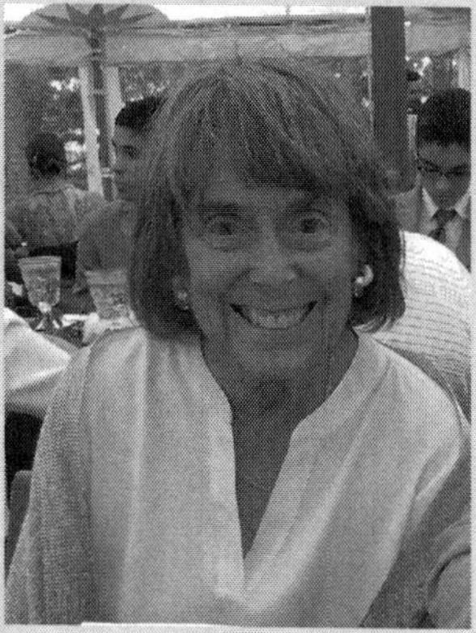

For Good
by Ann Reifman, PhD

I've heard it said
That people come into our lives
For a reason
Bringing something we must learn
And we are led to those
Who help us most to grow
If we let them
And we help them in return
But I don't know if I believe that's true
But I know I'm who I am today
Because I knew you
—by Stephen Schwartz from *Wicked*

THESE WORDS FROM WICKED RESONATE WITH ME. "I KNOW I'M WHO I AM TODAY" BECAUSE OF CERTAIN PEOPLE IN MY LIFE—MY PARENTS, MY SIBLINGS, PARTICULAR FRIENDS, SIGNIFICANT OTHERS, SPECIFIC TEACHERS, KIDS, GRANDKIDS AND OTHERS. Many patients have also made a difference. In this essay, I tell stories from two patients. Both stories come from years ago and from patients who carried the diagnosis of schizophrenia. One patient's story definitely had more impact on my life than the other, but both of these people made a difference.

I worked with "John" for years in a psychiatric hospital. (Those were the days when people could stay for years in a psychiatric hospital.) John was smart, kind, curious and also quite delusional at times. He believed he was God. John and I would often walk around the grounds of the hospital. I believe that for many people, especially people with psychosis, sitting and staring at each other in a therapy room is not always conducive to vulnerability, honesty and trust. Walking (or driving or sitting) side by side allows for people to feel less defensive and to be more open.

Sometimes when John and I walked, we would go across the street from the hospital to the grocery store or to MacDonalds. One time, we were sitting at MacDonalds about to eat. We had each ordered a Filet O'Fish. Just before I took my first bite, John held up his square fish patty and earnestly said, "This never swam in the sea." After a chuckle, I heard the wisdom of his words. Since 1982, thanks to John, I have never eaten a Filet O'Fish.

...

I worked with "George" for many years in my private psychotherapy practice. George was bright and often quite delusional; he thought he was a member of a famous rock band. Following the birth of my son, I had left psychiatric hospitals (primarily the National Institutes of Health or NIH) to have more control of my schedule. It was the first time in my career that I only worked in private practice. George and I usually met in my office, both of us sitting in the stress-free chairs that many therapists have...able to swivel to look at each other and able to turn away or anywhere in between; sometimes, we went for a walk. For years, George was the last patient I saw at the end of a long day.

> "Therapists do not say *Next* when inviting a patient from the waiting room."

One day, after about 10 years of full-time private practice, I went to the waiting room to get my last patient of the day (George) and heard myself say, "Next." NEXT! Therapists do not say *Next* when inviting a patient from the waiting room. Next was a word used for people coming to pick-up carryout orders, not for individuals coming to reflect on themselves. I was mortified that this word had come out of my mouth. Perhaps, I thought, George had not really heard me; perhaps he heard me, but would not say anything. He entered my office and we both sat down.

Suddenly, I heard George say, "Next?" Before I could respond, he said, "Something is not going right in your life." I thanked him for his clarity and for his honesty and told him that I wanted to think about his statement; we talked about how he felt about hearing the word and eventually we moved on to what else was happening in his life.

As soon as the session ended, I went to my husband's office. (He and I shared a psychotherapy suite and I knew he was waiting for me to drive home.) I told him what I had said when I went to invite my patient from the waiting room and what my patient had said. My husband responded, "I think it is time for you to return to NIH." The next day, I called old colleagues and within a couple months, I returned gleefully (and part time) to the psychiatric hospital.

"And we are led to those
Who help us grow
If we let them"

I might have lingered for years longer in fulltime private practice. I liked the freedom of this work and the patients who chose to come for therapy; I also appreciated the increased income compared to federal employment. However, I know I would have returned to a psychiatric hospital at some point. It is where I began my professional career; I loved the energy and mission of NIH; I reveled in the variety of tasks, from clinical work to research, writing, teaching and supervision; and I absolutely treasured working with seriously disturbed people as part of a team.

But without a doubt, I returned to NIH faster because of George, because I knew him, because I listened to his words, because I let myself be changed....for good.

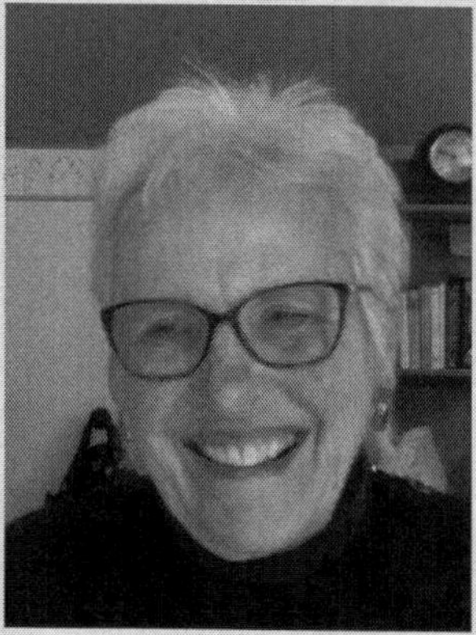

Looking Back
by Hallie Lovett, PhD

As best I can remember it would have been some time in 1975—an astonishing 50 years ago. The essential elements are as clear as day, although I'm sure I have hysterical amnesia for much of the event that took place. I was in the fourth year of my PhD program. Three years before, we had moved to the Washington DC area from Vermont newly married, so that I could attend graduate school. By now we had three and one-year old sons, a new house (and mortgage) and I was finishing up my internship at the Washington Veterans Administration Hospital and doing the research for my dissertation one day a week.

I was also deep into being, for the first time in my life, a therapy patient. Although I had a very positive transference to my therapist, there were obvious signs that some of my more reliable coping and defensive strategies were not helping. I was anxious, tired and seriously over-functioning. The first corners of my delayed dependency needs were coming into view, although this was to be a lifelong struggle.

"I could breathe again."

My therapist was a member of a weekly supervision group with Shelly Kopp. Kopp's membership in AAP was early and brief, even so, he had a very influential impact on many members of the Academy for over 20 years, including at least two presidents, until his death. Through his writing and roles as therapist and supervisor to many, Shelly was in the forefront of experiential psychotherapy. One of the innovative practices he developed was to ask members of the group to bring into the supervision session a patient with whom they felt "stuck" in the work.

I remember standing in the hallway on an upper floor of 5225 Connecticut Ave., NW looking out on the street waiting to be called into either the waiting room or the consultation room. I cannot remember one other person, in the group of about eight who met in that office, except for Shelly and, of course Jane, my therapist. This is noteworthy because I know for sure that I later became friends and colleagues with many of those in attendance that day. You might say I was a little nervous. I do remember

Shelly as warm, gracious and inviting, which surprised me because he had a reputation of being exceptionally direct and even confrontational. His welcome helped to relax me a bit. He asked both of us how we thought the therapy was going and where we thought our time together "might be bogged down in some way." I don't remember what I said, but I remember Jane telling everyone some of my history, including—to my horror and shame—that I was constipated as a child, along with its links to my demanding mother. After a short time, Shelly then encouraged the two of us to share with each other and with the larger group how we felt the present experience was going so far. I was mute, but Jane tried valiantly to elicit some kind of response from me, to get the interaction into some kind of dialogue between us. This went through a couple of iterations and I remember feeling completely on the spot, stymied, embarrassed, and unable to formulate any statement about anything, never mind how I was feeling. Then Shelly spoke directly to Jane and in the kindest but firmest of ways said, "Jane. Stop that. You're pushing her now."

I cannot exaggerate, recalling even now, fifty years on, the flow of relief and warmth, the sense of being seen and understood that I experienced in those fleeting few minutes after Shelly spoke to her. I could breathe again. I was flooded with a rush of understanding of how affect and language might come together in therapy—maybe for the first solid time, but thankfully not for the last.

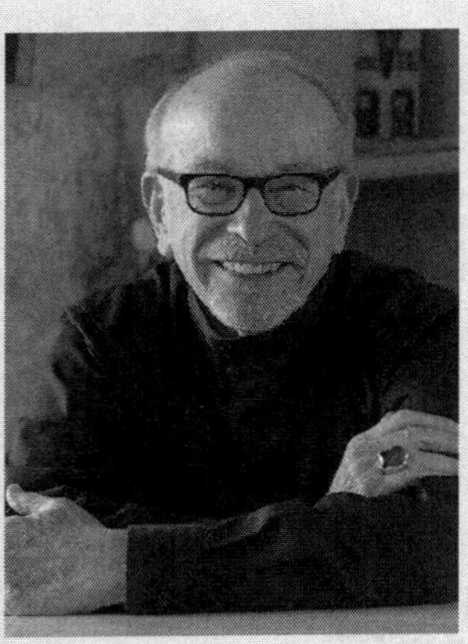

A Therapist Learns to Keep His Mouth Shut

by Murray Scher, PhD

As a new member, I had an opinion about everything and felt obligated to voice it at every community meeting. David Hawkins said to me, "You will have more influence if you say less." I did, and he was right.

I was in a group led by Vivian Guze. She outlined what she hoped would happen and then sat back. Silence followed for at least twenty minutes, it didn't just feel like twenty minutes, it was! Finally, someone spoke. Sol Rosenberg said, "Vivian you can tolerate silence longer than anyone I know." I thought, "I can do that." And I have.

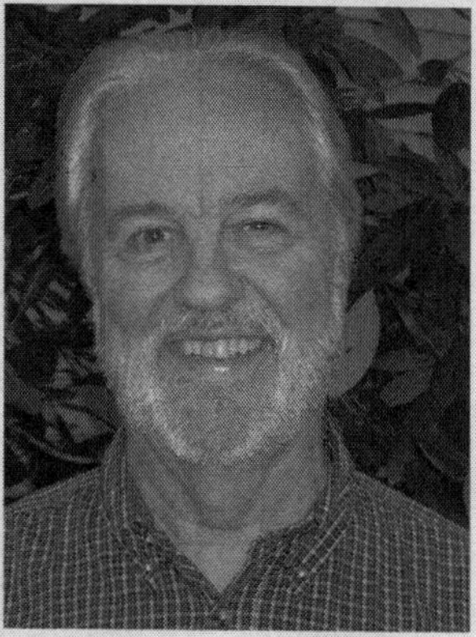

Finding AAP

by John Rhead, PhD

OVER 50 YEARS AGO NOW IN 1974, MY WIFE AND I FOUND OURSELVES IN A VERY COMPLICATED PLACE WITH REGARD TO HER EX-HUSBAND. I suggested to him that the three of us might try some therapy together. He told me that the only therapist he would consider seeing was the well-known and controversial Sheldon Kopp, whose books he had read. I called Dr. Kopp to make an appointment and he said that he would not touch our messy situation with a 10-foot pole. He gave me the names of two younger therapists he knew, Fred Klein and Barry Sternfeld, who he thought might be willing to take on our situation.

I called Barry, who also declined to see the three of us. He told me he would see me with my wife and also told me as a preliminary matter not to even mention his name to her ex-husband. My wife and I ended up doing some couples work and then I got into individual therapy with Barry. In his waiting room I frequently saw a journal entitled Voices, published by some—what seemed to me—wildly unorthodox organization called the American Academy of Psychotherapists. My individual work with Barry went on for quite a few years, during which I read many articles from Voices in his waiting room and ultimately got interested enough in AAP to join.

One day, when I was driving to my appointment with Barry, I burst into a gushingly emotional prayer of thanksgiving for having found him and for the work he and I had done together. Although I don't recall the exact words of my prayer, I think I was also expressing gratitude for having discovered AAP.

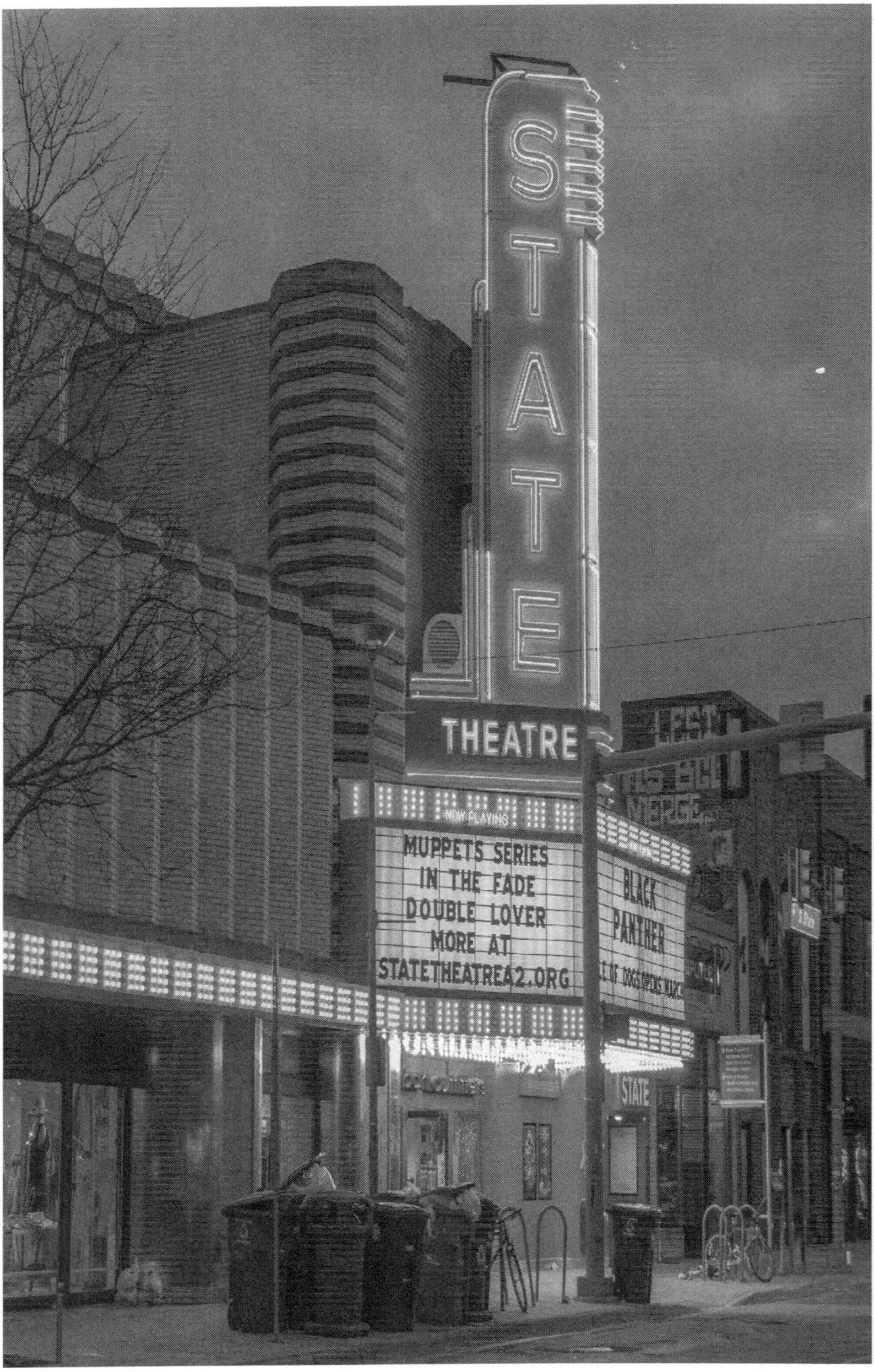

State Theatre by Jennifer Baumann

Ezra Farber

EZRA FARBER improves dog and human behavior in his dog training practice in Durham, North Carolina. He also creates interesting and bespoke objects for his friends with his 3D printer. *Farberezra@gmail.com*

Film Review

Thunderbolts

Group Connection versus Despair

OVER THE PAST FEW DECADES OF MARVEL SUPERHERO FILMS, I'VE FELT A WANING ENTHUSIASM FOR THE GENRE. As the scale and stakes depicted grew from terrestrial to galactic and the stable of heroic characters (who all needed their heroic moments on screen and rarely seemed to be in any actual danger) swelled to the dozens, the movies started to feel less grounded in humanity and more of a self-sustaining commercial franchise.

After all, what made superheroes so exciting to me as a kid leafing through a milk carton of my dad's worn and tattered comic books dating back to the 60s and 70s was not the "super," but the "human" and the characters in Thunderbolts feel all too human. They're depressed castoffs from the mainline world of heroes with shameful pasts and guilt from having been manipulated into doing terrible things. As Julia Louis-Dreyfus' shady CIA director puts it, they're "defective losers... antisocial tragedy in human form." They demonstrate familiar features of depression such as dismal self-esteem, fatalism drifting into inertia, and social withdrawal.

The movie isn't completely free of cliché. Of course, these losers need to come together and overcome their personal demons to protect civilians. But the way they do it is something I've rarely seen in a genre film. I hate to spoil the surprise, but as the film reaches its climax (the last act is where the meaningful emotional development of the movie takes place), they find themselves having to explore each other's chambers of guilt, shame, and trauma in an almost literal sense. They travel through these rooms by gazing into mirrors, a shared introspection that made me say out loud in the theater "oh, they're doing therapy!"

If you're looking for a psychologically convincing portrayal of depression, and an inspiring show of collective healing, or if you need a break from your real life or the problems of the real world, put *Thunderbolts* on your queue, and put super and human back together again.

"The film, poetry, art, and the therapist make possible the registration of horror. To be mastered, the unspeakable feelings evoked by the trauma must find communicable form, and a structure that gives them coherence and meaning."

—Janice Gump

Film Review

Emilia Pérez
Directed by Jacques Audiard

Bob Schulte

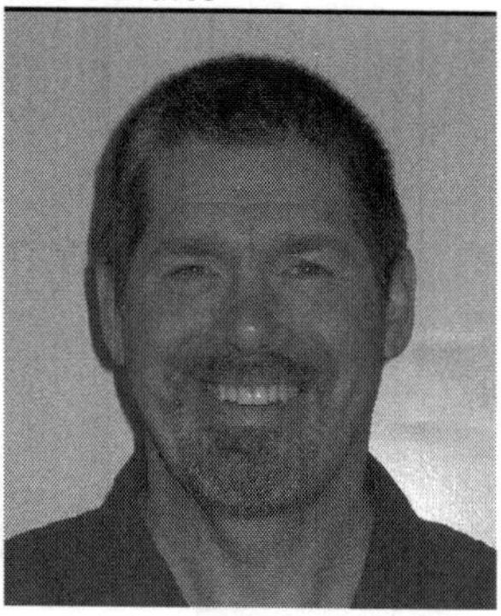

Bob Schulte, MSW is a psychotherapist in private practice in Alexandria, Virginia, offering individual and group therapy to adult patients. His former career as a stage director found expression in the Red Well Theater, a dramatic play reading group for and by therapists, designed to illuminate the impact of the social surround in and beyond the therapy group. Bob is a faculty member of the National Group Psychotherapy Institute at the New Washington School of Psychiatry. *bobgroup@aol.com*

"To thine own self be true" endures as a recognizable, loving admonition from a father preparing his beloved son to embark on a long journey in Shakespeare's Hamlet. Be honest with yourself. Live by your beliefs and values with fidelity. But the plot always thickens when the competing interests of others and the world writ large confront and confound those humble aspirations. Father Polonius' parting words of wisdom to son Laertes end with this final instruction: "And it must follow, as the night the day, thou canst not then be false to any man".

I introduce these universal tenets to serve as a frame for holding and considering the dual and dueling identities, hidden desires, secrets, deceits, rage, violence, traumatic losses, and yes, fidelity, compassion, and love, that are the stuff of Emilia Pérez, an award-winning, genre-defying, musical French film directed by Jacques Audiard.

The Plot Lines & Squiggles of Emilia Pérez

Manitas del Monte, husband, father, and a notorious drug cartel leader operating in Mexico City, is obsessed with completing gender-affirming surgery and transitioning to one Emilia Pérez. His dual aims are to escape legal troubles related to his criminal enterprise and even more desperately, to resolve a life-long gender dysphoria. Manitas seeks the assistance of a professionally frustrated lawyer Rita Moro Castro with a seductively large sum of money and some not-so-subtle intimidation as inducement. Rita accepts the offer. Together they engineer a believable death narrative for Manitas to guarantee his life-ever-after as Emilia. Leaving wife Jessi and two sons to grieve his lie alone was an emotional cost Manitas was willing to pay.

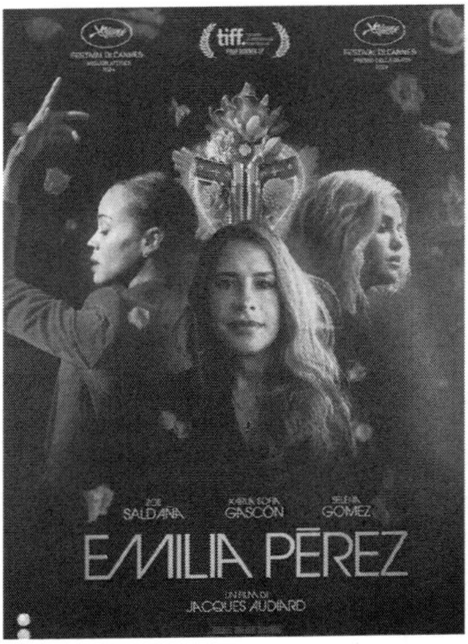

The eventual Ms. Pérez did not, however, plan to live without Jessi and their children for long. Emilia poses as a female distant cousin and becomes a live-in "Auntie" overseeing their collective lives. Emilia also sets out to make amends for the crimes she committed by championing the cause of those abducted and missing in Mexico, with Rita's savvy legal guidance and support. Emilia also makes a new romantic connection with Epifania, a Mexican widow whose missing husband had been found dead. Emilia's discovery of Jessi's prior marital infidelity with a local named Gustavo and her resumption of the affair with plans to marry him, ensures that Emilia Pérez will end like all Shakespearean tragedies. Not well.

A trans-woman actor, Karla Sofîa Gascón, plays both the male character Manitas and the trans-woman character Emilia, with dazzling effect and was recognized throughout the film industry's awards season for her outstanding performances. Counselor Moro Castro is portrayed by Zoe Saldaña, winning her a Supporting Oscar statue. Selena Gomez plays Jessi and Adriana Paz is cast as Epifania. The four female actors together as an ensemble received a rare collective Best Actress Award at the 2024 Cannes Film Festival.

While the release of the film generated praise and wide-ranging nominations and awards, criticism and controversy also followed. The movie was not well received by the public in Mexico and social activists and LGBTQ+ groups protested, advocating a boycott of the film. Objections included the casting of mostly non-Mexican actors with variable fluency speaking Spanish; shooting the film in the director's native France rather than Mexico where the action actually takes place; portraying trans people in what was felt to be stereotypical and demeaning ways; and a belief that the film minimizes unresolved and continuing disappearances of Mexicans and the suffering of their families at the hands of drug cartels and their crime bosses. Emilia's decision to become a social activist was felt by some to be made without the character giving sufficient recognition or atonement for Manitas' past criminal involvement. The film's themes of disrespect and exploitation are noteworthy parallels to these public reactions.

I offer two competing, yet strangely compatible interpretations of Emilia's motivation for becoming an activist in her new life. One is the aspirational desire for making amends that authentically align with her evolving identity, values, and life goals. The other more cynical interpretation would be of a narcissistic desire to build a high-profile, successful, and very comfortable new life, not unlike the one Emilia knew before. Manitas and Emilia are masterful at presenting themselves as something they are not, at least not completely, and getting their way. Emilia's deceits might be understood as evidence that Manitas' fatal flaw of ruthless self-interest survived the gender transition process and resides still in Emilia. Even in her dying moments, Emilia's touching revelation to Jessi of the truth of his/her/their identity might be both a calculation for

> "I encourage anyone planning to watch Emilia Perez for the first time to share the experience with trusted friends or colleagues."

sympathy to increase the chances of survival and a tender bid for reconnection and forgiveness, if only for a moment, before all is lost forever.

Clinical and Educational Relevance

"To listen is to accept." – Counselor Rita Moro Castro

I watched the film alone many times as a prelude to writing this review. My first take felt like sitting in a car during a hurricane! But with each subsequent viewing I came closer to finding the eye of the storm, more calmly registering new dimensions of the characters as their situations flew by, deepening my compassion for their existential plights, all the while falling in love with the rhythms and melodies of a native Spanish tongue that will never be mine to sing.

Emilia Pérez, appreciated as fundamentally a family melodrama, could be an interesting vehicle for therapists to examine some of the complex individual, couple, and family dynamics related to identity that enter our therapeutic spaces and to consider unconscious biases that might influence the treatment. As a fantasy exercise, imagine receiving one of the orphaned sons as a referral—at any point during the patient's life span. Many a ghost would inhabit that consulting room! What might that co-transference journey be like for you in the role of therapist?

A supervisor might ask a group of therapists-in-training to view the film and then explore these professionally relevant questions: "If by human nature I am predestined to have needs and desires inspiring various transitions throughout my life, can I imagine and explore some of those possibilities now, and consider the real or imagined challenges I might encounter? Could I do this in the presence of colleagues as part of my developmental journey as a therapist?"

I encourage anyone planning to watch Emilia Pérez for the first time to share the experience with trusted friends or colleagues, and collectively share your experience of the film with authenticity and mutual regard.

Erin McCarthy

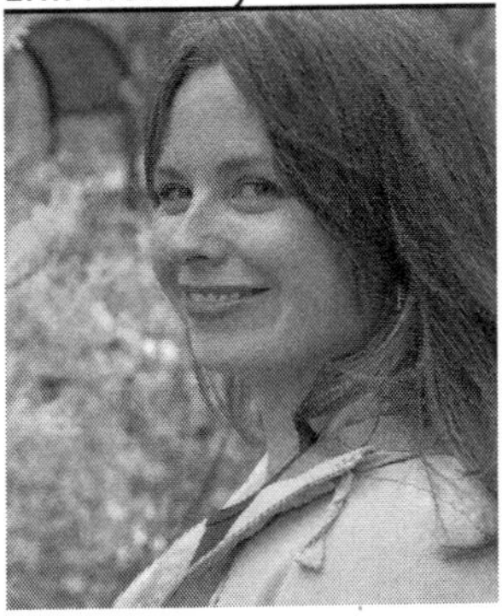

ERIN MCCARTHY, MSW, practices psychotherapy with adults, teenagers and groups. Her love of film and novels informs and colors her life and work. She maintains practices in Washington, DC, and Philadelphia, where she lives with her wife and four cats. *erin.elizabeth.mccarthy@gmail.com*

Voices is offering the option to listen to this article, enhancing accessibility and providing another way to engage with our content.
The following feature uses an automated voice, which may result in occasional errors in pronunciation, tone, or sentiment.

Book and Film Review

Small Things Like These, by Claire Keegan
Faber and Faber, 2021

Small Things LikeThese, 2024
Lionsgate Films

THIS PIECE WILL REVIEW CLAIRE KEEGAN'S 2021 NOVELLA *SMALL THINGS LIKE THESE* AND ITS FAITHFUL FILM ADAPTATION, RELEASED IN 2024. *Small Things Like These* could well apply to the number of words used in these works; Keegan's novella runs a spare 128 pages, enough to pass an afternoon, while the film, starring Cillian Murphy, communicates more in glances than in sentences. Murphy portrays Bill Furlong, an ordinary man torn between the dull consistency of the status quo and a stirring, personal dilemma. As readers and viewers, we are invited to spend a few days with Bill, his family and his flashbacks, as he finishes up the last coal deliveries of the year, just before Christmas 1985, coincidentally—the tail end of the year of my birth.

My Irish identity relies less on sketchy family history and more on an imagined and felt connection to this ancestral homeland. Dreaming of belonging, I named my childhood dog Shamrock and even briefly took on a traditional spelling of my name, Eireann. Recalling my visits to Ireland as a teen and young adult conjures up images of vast green vistas, cows and Celtic crosses dotting the landscape, a romantic pastoral view. My youthful grasping for idealized Irish roots lacked complexity and would have been well informed by the lived reality in Claire Keegan's novella and film adaptation. My fast forward tendencies, for example, might have been tempered by the lived experience of how in rural Ireland, then and now, one waits for the sheep to cross the road.

In *Small Things Like These,* one is transported to a small town that feels much older, that through tradition, poverty, and lack of exposure remains insulated from the larger world. Darkness and cold reveal the winter season, and the imagined landscapes of my personal vision are distant. Bill Furlong and his family live in the shadow of an imposing convent and school, a symbolic and literal representation of the immense influence of the hierarchy of the Catholic Church in Ireland. The convent runs a laundry service which requires coal for fuel, and Bill has to make a delivery from the coal yard. As he jiggles the lock to the yard, he notices that it is frozen solid and requires boiling hot water, "borrowed" from a neighbor, to yield. A similar process takes place in this narrative: Bill Furlong's frozen heart thaws and begins to beat, ever louder, as he is brought back to life by coming face to face with a girl and her suffering.

We meet Furlong in a frozen state, as he lives preoccupied by the shadow of his childhood. While outwardly 'functioning' as a father of five and owner of the town coal business, Furlong lives with intrapsychic wounds that haunt him, taking him far away from the daily churn of receipts, drop offs and complaints to an echoey place of emotional deprivation and confusion. Furlong shares this painful internal state with no one. It's clear the isolation is killing him, albeit slowly.

We learn that Bill's mother, unmarried and pregnant, was taken in by the Protestant landowner at the top of the hill before he was born. So Furlong has never been hungry, but has suffered profound emotional loss—the early death of his mother and the pain of not knowing his father. In the 2024 film, the viewer sees worry, pain, and longing pass over Furlong's face and remain unexpressed, locked down. In the absence of a soothing other, we see how Furlong has learned to soothe himself as well as the limitations of his powers of repression. In a house filled with laughter and caretaking, Furlong is a haunted, solitary man carrying a heavy load. He scrubs his hands raw upon returning home from the coal yard. He plunges his hands into icy water, numbing the disappointment.

Bill Furlong would be a great candidate for psychotherapy: haunted by his past, distant in his present life, disconnected from the happy chatter of his wife and kids. Unfortunately for Bill, Irish Catholicism doesn't quite align with psychotherapy on first or tenth glance, particularly in terms of access. Growing up in that milieu, I didn't know anyone who went to therapy or talked much about themselves in a deeper way. But it was at church that I experienced my first face-to-face encounter with confessing my sins and receiving comfort, an experience not too distant from the therapeutic encounter. I was terrified and intrigued by the prompt to tell Monsignor Ciaran O'Mearain, with his flexible, friendly face, what I had done wrong—meanness to my sibling, disrespect to my parents—and receive the reassuring balm of forgiveness. The confusion came, of course, when stories of ongoing sexual abuse by priests made headlines. Was the church a source for goodness, forgiveness and love? Or a hiding place for corruption and pedophilia?

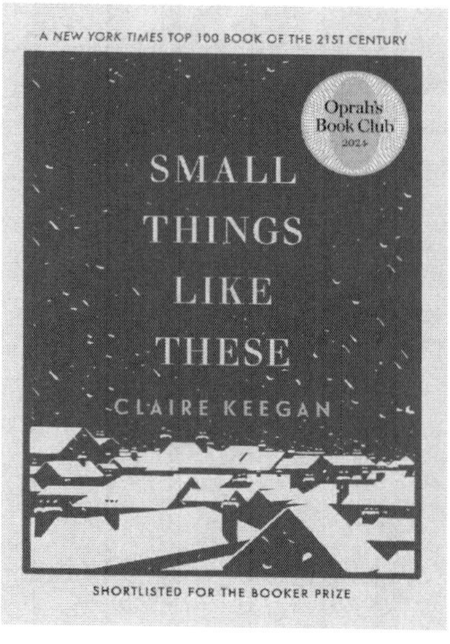

The prompt for self reflection and promise of forgiveness intrigued me—but I can't recall ever being prompted to explore why I might commit

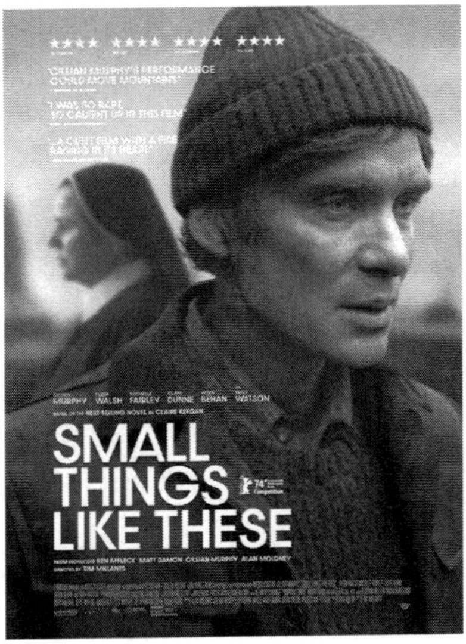

such sins or how I could do things differently. I recall a wish and a felt sense of cutting off my badness. Just stop doing that, and that's what God wants for you. In *Small Things Like These,* Keegan sketches a portrait of feminine obedience and punishment—Furlong's daughters study and help out in the coal yard. Other young girls, unwed mothers all, scrub the convent floor. Other women in the village are complicit in allowing the convent sisters' scheme of corruption to continue unfettered. Do what you're told, and you won't end up unlucky, and if anything happens to you, get over it because other people have it worse– you're lucky.

Bill Furlong has followed these guidelines and has ended up deadened inside. What breaks him from his dissociative isolation, though, is facing another human's suffering at the hands of those in power. Historical record reveals the troubling history of the Magdalene Laundries in Ireland, where young, vulnerable girls, abandoned by their families, were conscripted into working for room and board. It begins to dawn on Furlong that the laundry at the top of the hill may hide persistent and ongoing cruelty, with no accountability to ethics. Seeing this helpless girl, the face of this suffering stranger, gets him talking. Various town power brokers strongly encourage silence, or else—but Furlong will not be quieted.

The film and the book leave us wondering about what happens next; Keegan deliberately leaves us, and the central plot, with questions as the narrative concludes. But Bill's transformation is unmistakable, unmissable. As clinicians, we know that small things, more particularly the small things of psychotherapy, have the power to unlock states, memories and connection. A glance, a word, a moment, shared between two people, may spark a flame, a life force, that will continue burning, long after the encounter. I think the possibility of ignition, of generative energy, keeps me coming back to begin each small session, anew, ripe with possibility of what could be. While it may be cold and dark, together, we can keep the fire burning.

Future Issues

PLEASE PARDON OUR DUST...AS *VOICES* NAVIGATES SOME TRANSITION. Timelines and Calls for Papers beyond the 2026 issue are not yet ready for publication, so watch our website for updates between issues.

https://www.aapweb.com/voices-journal/call-for-papers/

Call for Papers

Direct questions and submissions to Jonathan Farber *Jonathan.Farber@gmail.com.*

See Submission Guidelines on the AAP website: **www.aapweb.com** or in any issue of *Voices*

Subscribe to Voices

The American Academy of Psychotherapists invites you to be a part of an enlightening journey into...

VOICES

Voices is a uniquely rewarding publication providing a meeting ground with other experienced psychotherapists. A theme-oriented journal, *Voices* presents personal and experiential essays by therapists from a wide range of orientations. Each issue takes you on an intimate journey through the reflections of therapists as they share their day-to-day experiences in the process of therapy. *Voices'* contributors reveal insights inherent in our lives, our culture and our society.

As a subscriber, you'll have the opportunity to experience contributions from noted luminaries in psychotherapy. Using various styles from articles to poems, *Voices* is interdisciplinary in its focus, reflecting the aims and mission of its publisher, the American Academy of Psychotherapists.

VOICES **SUBSCRIPTION**

Please start my one-year subscription to AAP's journal *Voices* at $65 for individuals PDF only; $85 for individuals PDF & print copy. Institutional subscriptions may be reserved directly through the AAP office or through the traditional subscription agencies at $249 per year. *Voices* is published electronically and is delivered to your email address as an ePublication.

Address ....

City .... State .... ZIP ....

Telephone ....

Email ....

☐ My check made payable to AAP Voices is enclosed.
☐ Please charge to my credit card, using the information I have supplied below:

Form of payment: ☐ Master Card ☐ Visa

Account # .... Expiration: ....

Signature ....

Address all orders by mail to:

The Executive Director of AAP is LeAnna Hamer and her email address for all business inquiries (subscriptions, change of address, etc.) is: *aapexecdirector@gmail.com*, or check the *Voices* menu at AAPweb.com. The postal address for AAP is: P.O. Box 3220, Kingsport, TN 37664.

Guidelines for Contributors

Voices: The Art and Science of Psychotherapy, is the journal of the American Academy of Psychotherapists. Written by and for psychotherapists and healing professionals, it focuses on therapists' personal struggles and growth and on the promotion of excellence in the practice of psychotherapy. The articles are written in a personalized voice rather than an academic tone, and they are of an experiential and theoretical nature that reflects on the human condition.

Each issue has a central theme as described in the call for papers. Manuscripts that fit this theme are given priority. Final decision about acceptance must wait until all articles for a particular issue have been reviewed. Articles that do not fit into any particular theme are reviewed and held for inclusion in future issues on a space available basis.

Articles. See a recent issue of *Voices* for general style. Manuscripts should be double-spaced in 12 point type and no longer than 4,000 words (about 16 to 18 pages). Do not include the author's name in the manuscript, as all submissions receive masked review by two or more members of the Editorial Review Board. Keep references to a minimum and follow the style of the *Publication Manual of the American Psychological Association,* 5th ed.

Submit via email, attaching the manuscript as a Word document file. Send it to Jonathan Farber at *JonathanFarber@gmail.com.* Put "Voices" in the email's subject line, and in the message include the author's name, title and degree, postal address, daytime phone number, manuscript title, and word count. Please indicate for which issue of *Voices* the manuscript is intended.

If a manuscript is accepted, the author will be asked to provide a short autobiographical sketch (75 words or less) and a photograph that complies with technical quality standards outlined in a PDF which will be sent to you.

Neither the editorial staff nor the American Academy of Psychotherapists accepts responsibility for statements made in its publication by contributors. We expect authors to make certain there is no breach of confidentiality in their submissions. Authors are responsible for checking the accuracy of their quotes, citations, and references.

Poetry. We welcome poetry of high quality relevant to the theme of a particular issue or the general field of psychotherapy. Short poems are published most often.

Book and Film Reviews. Reviews should be about 500 to 750 words, twice that if you wish to expand the material into a mini-article.

Visual Arts. We welcome submissions of photographs or art related to the central theme for consideration. Electronic submissions in JPEG or TIFF format are required. If you would like to submit images, please request the PDF of quality standards from Kim Leaird at *kimleaird@me.com* or find it on www.aapweb.com. Images are non-returnable and the copyright MUST belong to the submitting artist.

Copyright. By submitting materials to *Voices* (articles, poems, photos or artwork), the author transfers and consents that copyright for that article will be owned by the American Academy of Psychotherapists, Inc.

Vision Statement

Our vision is to be the premier professional organization where therapeutic excellence and the use of self in psychotherapy flourish.

Mission Statement

The mission of the American Academy of Psychotherapists is to invigorate the psychotherapist's quest for growth and excellence through authentic interpersonal engagement.

Core Values

- Courage to risk and willingness to change
- Balancing confrontation and compassion
- Commitment to authenticity with responsibility
- Honoring the individual and the community

Full Membership

Full Membership in the Academy requires a doctoral or professional degree in one of the following mental health fields: psychiatry, clinical or counseling psychology, social work, pastoral counseling, marriage and family therapy, counseling, or nursing, and licensure which allows for the independent practice of psychotherapy.

- Specific training in psychotherapy with a minimum of 100 hours of supervision.
- At least one year of full-time post graduate clinical experience (or the equivalent in part-time experience) for doctoral level applicants, at least two years for others.
- A minimum of 100 hours of personal psychotherapy.

A person who does not fulfill the above requirements but who is able to document a reasonable claim for eligibility, such as a distinguished contributor to the field of psychotherapy, may also be considered for full membership.

Other Categories of Membership

In the interest of promoting the development of experienced psychotherapists, one category of associate membership is offered for those with the intent of becoming full members. These members will be working with a mentor as they progress to Full Membership.

Associate Membership

- has completed a relevant professional degree
- is currently practicing psychotherapy under supervision appropriate to the licensure
- has recommendations from at least three faculty, supervisors, and/or Academy members
- has completed or is actively engaged in obtaining 100 hours of personal psychotherapy
- agrees to work with an Academy member mentor
- may be an associate for no more than five years

Student Affiliate

For students currently enrolled in a graduate degree program. Application includes acceptable recommendations from two faculty supervisors or Academy members.

For information regarding membership requirements or to request an application, contact the Central Office. Membership information and a printable application form are also available on the Academy's Web site, www.aapweb.com.

Executive Office

LeAnna Hamer, *Executive Director*
P.O. Box 3220
Kingsport, TN 37664

Made in the USA
Monee, IL
15 June 2026

54243522R00077